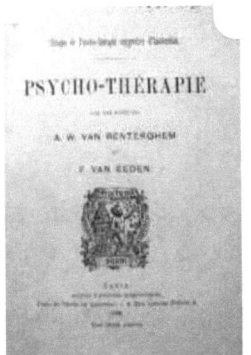

TRANSLATED FROM THE FRENCH BY

Stephen Wilson

LAMAD VAV PRESS

Oxford

Lamad Vav Press, Oxford

Psycho-Therapy

Translation © Stephen Wilson 2019

All rights reserved

This book is sold subject to the condition that it shall not by way of trade or otherwise, be lent, resold, hired out or otherwise circulated without the publisher's prior consent in any form of binding or cover other than that in which it is published and without a similar condition, including this condition, being imposed on the subsequent purchaser.

First published in French under the title *Psycho-therapie*, © Société d'èditions scientifiques, 1894.

For Chaitan Haldipur

# PSYCHO-THERAPY

******

Statistical communications,

New clinical observations

******

## REPORT

*of the results obtained in the* **Amsterdam Suggestive Psycho-therapy Clinic**, *during the second period* **1889—1893;**

### BY DOCTORS

A.W. VAN RENTERGHEM and F. VAN EEDEN.

PARIS

SOCIÉTÉ D'ÈDITIONS SCIENTIFIQUES,

Place de l'Ecole de médecine. — 4. Rue Antoine Dubois, 4.

1894 All rights reserved.

# TABLE OF CONTENTS

Preface.

Introduction.

General summary of statistics (covering all cases treated from 5 May 1887 to 30 June 1893).

Clinical observations.

A. GROUP I. ORGANIC CONDITIONS OF THE NERVOUS SYSTEM

Obs.1.Syphilitic hemiplegia and epilepsy; mixed treatment; slight improvement.

Obs.2.Transverse myelitis (?) complicated with hysteria; marked improvement.

Obs. 3. Multiple sclerosis; small improvement.

Obs. 4. Left hemiplegia, following apoplexy; improvement.

A. GROUP II. GRAND NEUROSES

Obs.5. Severe hysteria, improvement by hypnotic suggestion. Cure of all symptoms by prolonged sleep. Relapse.

Obs. 6. Virile hysteria. Chronic cephalgia. Cure.

Obs. 7. Symptoms of round ulcer of the stomach followed by sciatica. Cure by hypnotic suggestion. Diverse hysterical symptoms cured as and when they presented during the course of five consecutive years by the same treatment.

Obs. 8. Uncontrollable vomiting in a hysteric. Cure.

Obs.9.Uncontrollable vomiting in a hysteric, resistant to the usual medication, cured by one session of suggestion.

Obs. 10. Vomiting of food in a hysteric, cure.

Obs. 11. Hysterical paraplegia dating back 12 years, cured by suggestion. relapse after 4 years. New cure.

Obs. 12 Functional paraplegia? (Abasia,astasia) resistant to various treatments and abandoned as incurable; notable permanent improvement by psychotherapy.

Obs. 13. Hystero-epilepsy; cure.

Obs. 14 Hystero-epilepsy, improvement obtained through suggestion; relapse resulting from premature suspension of treatment.

Obs. 15. Epileptic fits in a hysteric. Cure achieved in a single session of suggestion.

Obs. 16. Epileptic fits in a hysterical man. Cure.

Obs. 17. Hystero-epilepsy, tic douloureux, cure.

Obs. 18. Virile hysteria. Overwhelming anxiety state in a patient while carrying out his professional duties, impossibility of continuing his employment. cure in several sessions.

Obs. 19. Severe nervous attacks of a hysterical type; cure.

Obs. 20. Anorexia, insomnia, persistent hiccup in a hysteric. Notable improvement. relapse after 9 months. resumption of treatment followed by cure.

Obs. 21. Continuous laryngeal chorea in a hysteric, persisting for two years, cured by hypnotic suggestion.

Obs. 22. Trembling and fits of eructation in a hysteric. Cure.

Obs. 23. Different functional problems presenting over the course of three consecutive years in an hysteric, cured by suggestion.

Obs. 24. Tinnitus and diverse noises in the ears; cure by hypnotic suggestion.

Obs. 25. Fits of anger and bad humour in a hysteric. Cure by hypnotic suggestion.

Obs. 26. Hysterical anaemia, chronic headaches for four years, refractory to medical treatment, cured by psycho-therapy.

Obs. 27. Spontaneous somnambulism, cured by one session of suggestion.

Obs. 28. Obsessive erotic dreams, menorrhagia. Curettage of the womb. Periods become normal. Nervous symptoms persist. Bilateral oophorectomy. Aggravation of nervous state. Marked improvement through hypnotic suggestion.

Obs. 29. Haemoptysis apparently hysterical, resistant to medical treatment, cured by hypnotic suggestion.

Obs. 30. Anxiety state causing inability to sing and lack of effort to memorise in a hysterical pupil of the conservatoire, cured by hypnotic suggestion.

Obs. 31. Cerebral neurasthenia. headaches. Inability to continue his studies in a student. Cure.

Obs. 32. Neurasthenic symptoms cured by hypnotic suggestion.

Obs. 33. Severe neurasthenia, dating back ten years, refractory to all treatment. Notable and persistent improvement thanks to treatment by suggestion continued and lasting more than 4 years.

Obs. 34. Severe neurasthenia; notable improvement. relapse.

Obs. 35. Neurasthenia. Motor asthenia predominant. notable improvement.

Obs. 36. Severe neurasthenia. Motor asthenia predominant. Notable and persistent improvement of the principal phenomena.

Obs. 37. Mixed form of two grand neuroses: hysteria and neurasthenia. Notable persistent improvement.

Obs. 38. Hystero-neurasthenia. Marked improvement obtained by psychotherapy.

Obs. 39. Constipation giving rise to nervous attacks of a neurasthenic nature, in a hereditary predisposition. Mixed treatment by medicines and suggestion. Cure.

Obs. 40. Neurasthenic hypochondria, cure.

Obs. 41. Obsessive idea. Cure by psycho-therapy.

Obs. 42. Insomnia accompanied by fear of going mad in a neurasthenic; marked improvement.

Obs. 43. Resistant insomnia, agoraphobia, suicidal thoughts. Marked improvement through suggestion.

Obs. 44. Fear of open spaces, horror of heights, nosophobia improved by psycho-therapy.

Obs. 45. Nervous symptoms, obsessional ideas triggered by pregnancy in a hereditary predisposition; cured by hypnotic suggestion.

Obs. 46. Obsessive idea suppressed by hypnotic suggestion.

Obs. 47. Nervous tremor, obsessional idea. Cure by hypnotic suggestion.

Obs. 48. Various neuropathic troubles: insomnia, depression, nosophobia, in a hereditarily predisposed person. Cure of symptoms by hypnotic suggestion.

Obs. 49. Melancholia, obsessive ideas, suicidal and homicidal impulses. Cure obtained by the suggestive method.

Obs. 50. Nervous dyspepsia, refractory to different drug treatments, cured by suggestion in a waking state.

A. GROUP III. MENTAL ILLNESSES

Obs. 51. Nervous attacks; night terrors in a hereditarily predisposed child. Very marked improvement.

Obs. 52. Moral insanity, temporary improvement.

Obs. 53. Moral insanity, nocturnal incontinence of urine, very marked improvement.

Obs. 54. Lypemania. Obsessional compulsions, temporary improvement.

Obs. 55. Chronic melancholia, failure of the suggestive method.

Obs. 56. Melancholia with insight, mixed treatment.

Obs. 57. Melancholia without delusions, notable improvement.

Obs. 58. Lypemania, chronic constipation, cure by hypnotic suggestion.

Obs. 59. Periodic dipsomania, cure by hypnotic suggestion. relapse.

Obs. 60. Periodic dipsomania. Cure lasting three years. Relapse.

Obs. 61. Alcoholism cured by suggestion.

Obs. 62. Alcoholic habits. Cure.

## A. GROUP IV. NEUROPATHIC CONDITIONS

Obs. 63. Bronchial asthma, cured by hypnotic suggestion.

Obs. 64. Bronchial asthma, decided improvement.

Obs. 65. Periodic bronchial asthma, hemicrania. Cure of the asthma, notable improvement in the migraine.

Obs. 66. Asthmatic hay fever, cure by hypnotic suggestion.

Obs. 67. Asthmatic hay fever, notable improvement.

Obs. 68. Asthmatic hay fever, cure.

Obs. 69. Recent onset of stuttering in a boy, cured by hypnotic suggestion.

Obs. 70. Stuttering and spasmodic facial tic, very marked improvement, continuation of treatment.

Obs. 71. Habitual masturbation; improvement.

Obs. 72. Diurnal and nocturnal incontinence of urine. Periodic cephalgia. cure.

Obs. 73. Nocturnal incontinence of urine. Cure.

Obs. 74. Urinary incontinence, cured by hypnotic suggestion. relapse followed by definitive cure.

Obs. 75. Urinary incontinence, cure.

Obs. 76. Nocturnal incontinence of urine, failure.

Obs. 77. Nocturnal incontinence of urine, cure.

Obs. 78. Nocturnal incontinence of urien, treatment by hypnotic suggestion, result unknown.

Obs. 79. Nocturnal incontinence of urine, cure.

Obs. 80. Habitual nocturnal incontinence of urine, cure.

Obs. 81. Nocturnal incontinence of urine; dubious result.

Obs. 82. Incontinence of urine and faeces day and night; improvement.

Obs. 83. Incontinence of urine night and day. Failure.

Obs. 84. Nocturnal incontinence of urine, chorea, cure.

Obs. 85. Incontinence of urine day and night. Cure.

Obs. 86. Nocturnal incontinence of urine, marked improvement.

Obs. 87. Nocturnal incontinence of urine, decided improvement.

Obs. 88. Incontinence of urine, cure.

Obs. 89. Incontinence of urine. Failure.

Obs. 90. Incontinence of urine day and night, cure.

Obs. 91. Incontinence of urine day and night. Notable improvement.

A. GROUP V. NEURALGIAS PAINS CRAMPS

Obs. 92. Habitual cephalgia, cure.

Obs. 93. Habitual cephalgia, cure.

Obs. 94. Spasmodic functional contraction of the hands. Cure.

Obs. 95. Sacro-lumbar neuralgia, cure by suggestion in the waking state in a single session.

Obs. 96. Chronic sciatica for six years, cure.

Obs. 97. Chronic sciatica for six years, hysterical symptoms, cure.

Obs. 98. Tic douloureux dating back 25 years. very decided improvement.

Obs. 99. Tic douloureux dating back 3 years. Neurectomy. persistence of neuralgia. cure by suggestion. Relapse. New Cure.

Obs. 100. Right prosopalgia, cure in three suggestive sessions.

Obs. 101. Tic douloureux for one year, cure by hypnotic suggestion.

Obs. 102. Habitual cephalgia and spasmodic tic, notable improvement.

Obs. 103. Gastro-intestinal neuralgia. Unilateral ovariectomy. Persistence of the neuralgia. decided improvement as a result of psycho-therapy.

Obs. 104. Gastralgia linked in all probability to a scarred stomach ulcer, cure.

Obs. 105. Multiple chronic neuralgias in a hysteric, refractory to various treatments, cured by hypnotic suggestion.

Obs. 106. Anal prolapse in a 5-year- old child, cure by hypnotic suggestion.

B. GROUPS VI&VII. ILLNESSES OF DIVERSE ORGANS AND SYSTEMS (OTHER THAN THE NERVOUS SYSTEM)

B. GROUP VIII. ANAEMIA MENSTRUAL ABNORMALITIES

C. GROUP IX. SURGICAL ANAESTHESIA

Obs. 107. Complete rupture of the perineum dating back several years. Radical operation without notable pain under the influence of suggestion without sleep.

Obs. 108. Laparotomy, total removal of the uterus and its appendices. surgical anaesthesia obtained with a small dose of chloroform together with hypnotic suggestion.

Obs. 109. Painless extraction of a tooth. Suggestive analgesia.

Obs. 110. Analgesia by suggestion; painless extraction of a tooth.

## Preface

In the six years between 1887 and 1893, Van Renterghem and Van Eeden treated more than a thousand patients in their Amsterdam suggestive psychotherapy clinic. This book summarises the results of their work. It was addressed to the medical profession and clearly intended to provide an evidential base which would justify the use of the method. But it also had a larger purpose, to counter prevailing materialistic conceptions of the human mind and to make the case for a reconsideration of vitalism. In demonstrating the influence of suggested ideas over both psychological and somatic processes, they highlighted the inadequacy of mechanistic explanations.

Both authors allied themselves to the therapeutic methods of Ambroise August Liébeault and Hyppolite Bernheim whom they had visited at Nancy, France. But they were at pains to distinguish what they were doing from the dramatic hypnotic séances given by Jean-Martin Charcot in Paris, and the dubious, but undeniably popular, activities of various stage-hypnotists, magnetists and mountebanks. Charcot thought suggestibility was pathognomonic of hysteria. He was more interested in using hypnotism to induce symptoms such as anaesthesia or paralysis, and thus clinch a diagnosis, than in its application for therapeutic purposes; whereas the Nancy school believed that suggestibility was distributed to varying degrees in the general population and could be harnessed for the benefit of patients. For this reason Van Renterghem and Van Eeden preferred the use of the term psycho-therapy.

Although Van Renterghem had developed a reputation for working miracles, the wariness of orthodox medicine meant that patients were frequently referred to the clinic as a last resort rather than a first port of call. Publication of these case-histories and the accompanying statistics was meant to reverse this process, demonstrate the wide range of medical conditions for which suggestion was an appropriate treatment, and introduce it into the realm of medical respectability.

By the time this book was published Van Eeden had lost interest in individual psycho-therapy, preferring to devote himself to literature and social reform. He did meet Freud in 1914 (who had himself moved away from his initial infatuation with hypnotism) and flirted briefly with psychoanalysis but turned against it, he went on to become much more interested in metaphysical speculation, spiritualism and religion. By contrast Van Renterghem later enthusiastically embraced psychoanalysis and in 1917 co-founded the Dutch branch of the International Psychoanalytic Association, of which he was elected the first president. He continued to practice psychotherapy until well into his ninth decade.[1]

In making this translation I have concentrated on the more than one hundred clinical observations which not only portray their subjects in an extraordinarily vivid way but also contribute to a convincing social history of the time. The colonial attitude and language which occurs when the authors talk about "the force of regeneration being greater in uncivilised people" is offensive today but also of its time.

The book contains 47 pages of detailed statistical tables, no doubt intended to impress medical colleagues, which break down the results into diagnostic category, age and sex of patient, level of hypnosis achieved and degree of

---

[1]* Bulhof, I. From Psychotherapy to psychoanalysis: Frederik Van Eeden and Albert Willem Van Renterghem, *J. History of the Behavioural Sciences,* 17 (1981) 209-221.

improvement obtained. I need to be forgiven for omitting all but one of these, which is a general summary, but the interested reader can find the rest in the original text.[2] By way of compensation I have included extra footnotes marked with an asterisk, not in the original text, wherever I have come across an abstruse medical term, a Latin or Greek tag, or anything else which I think might need explaining. I have also substituted full stops for semi-colons in many passages written in the telegraphic style of medical notes and sometimes failed to resist editing a redundant repetition which interfered with the flow of the text.

---

[2] See. https://www.biusante.parisdescartes.fr/histoire/medica/resultats/index.php?do=livre&cote=50553.

# INTRODUCTION

In presenting our latest findings to the medical public, we believe we have to underline once again the considerable significance for medicine in general which the success of a methodical psycho-therapy, understood in the widest sense of the word, necessarily entails.

Indeed it would appear that psycho-therapy, not simply "hypnotism" but the more general art of curing by psychological means, is already achieving satisfactory results despite the short duration of its existence as a methodical branch of medicine. Notwithstanding its as yet incomplete development, and so many contrary forces, it is not only maintaining its position but gaining increasing numbers of proponents. Clearly it is not simply a matter of adding one more routine tool to the therapeutic armamentarium. There is a need for fundamental reconsideration, indeed revision of basic therapeutic principles.

If the vast majority of scientists and academic physicians were, *a priori,* not expecting such favourable results, if they declared them in principle not only unlikely but even impossible, and if they denied them, disavowed them and judged them unbelievable and unacceptable despite the factual evidence, we can only conclude that these results fly in the face of received wisdom.

It is true and has been repeated ad nauseam that the ability of psychological factors to influence morbid symptoms has been well known for a long time, and that we have occasionally been able to judiciously put that knowledge to use with good effect. But it is also true that we have underestimated their power, that we have no in depth experience, and that psychological means have been applied with a lack of confidence and a lack of concern for specific indications or any particular method.

If today's medicine has approved and even recommended the use of psychological treatment in exceptional cases, it is far from applying it systematically. It certainly doesn't acknowledge the fact, which has now become a certainty, that a psycho-therapeutic system of treatment can be utilised almost exclusively in a domain embracing the totality of the neuroses[3] and psycho-neuroses, and even more widely, and that the results obtained are equivalent to or even surpass those obtained when following current best practice.

If one puts a different interpretation on the statistical and casuistic publications that have appeared in France, Sweden, Holland, England and Germany over the last five years, it

---

[3] * In 1894 this term denoted physical (psychosomatic) as well as mental conditions.

seems to us beyond doubt that a wider range of conditions could be treated with benefit using almost exclusively psychological means, while only having recourse to chemical, physical and electrical agents in exceptional circumstances; principally the neuropathies — it is true — but including the most difficult cases. It is clear that we can no longer explain this success by attributing it on the one hand to the enthusiastic blindness of doctors lacking a critical faculty, and on the other hand to the deference and credulity of the general public. Even so, the phenomenon is remarkable enough to raise doubts as to the validity of all the research published by doctors, so often lacking in detail, and appearing profusely in the journals.

It is timely to observe that medicine is still not very advanced when it sees the triumphs of homeopathy arising less from the effect of homeopathic remedies than the elimination of allopathic ones. Does psycho-therapy likewise have an insignificant or very little effect? One might conclude that we could do without the vast majority of usual remedies in our practice without suffering any particularly harmful consequences. A conclusion which, quite honestly, isn't immaterial when one considers just how damaging overprescribing can be.

At the end of the day it might be suggested that thaumaturges and charlatans have demonstrated since time immemorial that a perfectly chimerical medicine can attract a large number of adherents, and that this can easily be explained by the wildly exaggerated stories of cure put about by certain quasi-healers, and by the attraction of the "new" which persuades the inevitable contingent of incurables to have one last try; so that there is no need to postulate another more general psychological factor. We must reply to this argument that these cases accumulate as a result of unmet need or some analogous factor, and that their numbers are scarcely sustained for more than a few months in the same place if the therapeutic agent is not an effective one.

We ourselves could clearly distinguish between the first flush of patients —at the opening of our psycho-therapeutic clinic — people longing for something new and wonderful, attracted by overblown stories and gossip; and the ordinary, down-to-earth, normal clientele, rather more embarrassed than driven by popular opinion and clamour, and seeking treatment on the basis of the known undeniable results.

The first kind of patient came, partly motivated by curiosity or in the expectation of finally getting their hands on a miraculous remedy which would instantaneously relieve them of chronic or incurable ills. Mistaken in their expectation, these people failed to return after one or two sessions. In the beginning there were many of these visitors, but after a short time they became rare and gave way to the type of ordinary patient who doesn't expect miracles and comes for advice and guidance.

We dare to suppose however, that most doctors understand the power of suggestion sufficiently not to wish to conflate a psycho-therapeutic success with the success of a nihilistic therapy. They would accept that suggestion constitutes the therapeutic agent here just as it does with charlatans, secret remedies, miraculous springs, somnambulists etc.

But if one accepts that proposition we emphatically insist once again, that one examine the conclusions which follow from it. It is not sufficient to note that the existence of such quacks and their dupes, so many of whom are enemies and detractors of official medicine, now acquires a more reasonable and worthy justification than that of simple bad faith, stupidity or prejudice. There is an urgent need to take advantage of such a change of perspective. If one contents oneself with saying to those people healed by illegitimate means: "Fine, it's suggestion that has cured you!" they have a right to reply: "So why, hasn't official medicine cured us by suggestion?" And if one is convinced that this medical agent is being widely applied by incompetents, without knowing what they're doing, without any knowledge of the diseases they're treating, lacking discernment and without control, sometimes even unconscionably, isn't it time to take it out of their hands?

And that can only be done by first adopting a better way of working. In default of this condition the public will continue — despite legal proscriptions — to hold incompetents more competent than qualified doctors.

Without doubt doctors have for too long underestimated the judgement of the public, and placed too much emphasis on their own views. It has been demonstrated over the years, even centuries, that things observed and applied with advantage by laymen went unrecognised by gentlemen of the art. That these laymen didn't understand the finer details is of no consequence, it wasn't their business. But they got results, and medicine which laughed for such a long time and complained about their stupidity, must now following its obstinate opposition, acknowledge their rightness. To stay up on our high-horse gets us nowhere; it's a matter of recognising a mistake and correcting it by being more careful in future and scrupulously revising the principles that rendered this scorn possible.

The cause of the error resides in the double character of medical science which seeks to marry pure science with practical utility. Like the exact sciences it is inclined to follow an ideal course and never be rushed by utilitarian motives, to build its system in a rational and consistent way. However, its sphere of practical activity forces it to deviate from this principle. It has to act and make decisions even when it is not possible to be strictly scientific.

In effect, medicine serves two masters, science and suffering humanity. We most often link them together, we like to think that they go hand in hand, but it isn't always the case. Pure science would be very embarrassed if it always had to aim for a practical goal. It can take credit for making possible, even indirectly, innumerable practical applications, thanks to a strict adherence to its principles. But in its own workings it dares not pay attention to or aim at these applications. It serves a single master, and this ideal character is its pride and its power.

To avoid falling into error, there is an urgent need for the doctor to continue to clearly distinguish and attend to the dual function of his role. It is only in the laboratory that he can and must follow a purely scientific system. In the clinic it behoves him to take a different attitude. He must always understand that medical practice at the bedside is only rarely based on solid inductive scientific evidence and that it more often departs from this in favour of the nebulous spheres of empiricism, opinion and supposition. He has to understand that the sense of positiveness and certainty and the "a priori" permitted in the laboratory, are out of place at the bedside and must be replaced by an open-minded expectation without prejudgement of events, and by an acceptance of all the facts, however inexplicable they may be.

But this hasn't happened. Medicine believed itself able to judge, as if it knew what the mind could and couldn't do. So it hasn't paid sufficient attention to the seemingly inexplicable facts. It has put itself in the wrong vis-a-vis the lay public and failed to accomplish its mission. It seems necessary to insist on this once again because there are signs that we still have no guarantee against a repetition.

Speaking of what the mind can and cannot do, we need to enlarge on what we've said, as we will inevitably come up against psychologists who think their inexact or superficial theories permit them to conclude that it can do nothing.[4] From the practical point of view we also have little against the theory which states that a man who wants something isn't bothered by determinist conclusions that he isn't really choosing. Indeed it is not freedom but the opposite of

---
[4] German psychologists of the Wundt school: Lange, Ziehen et al.

freedom which seems to be the case. An appearance which we cause by confusing our mental constructs, which are indeed unfree — with reality, in which we find ourselves embedded as an active participant.

By the same type of error in reasoning we come to confuse the mind with consciousness and to consider it an appendage of our being immune to all investigation, whose active power is negligible, when in fact it should rather be thought of as a quality arising from the integration of diverse parts of our being whose active power nobody doubts.

What we understand by mind (Ψυχη)[5] is thus that part of our being which is open to direct or introspective observation.

It is worth noting again that there is as much, even more reason to treat the unconscious part of ourselves — our body, as enigmatic, impenetrable, inexplicable and non-autonomous, as the conscious part — our mind. Since we never perceive the body directly, but only through the intermediary of the mind; we get to the former by inference and thus it always has a rather hypothetical character. In many people's eyes this seems a paradoxical and excessive speculation. It is however a simple truth, long known, but

---
[5] *Psyche.

lost from sight since the extent and solidity of our system of natural sciences made us confuse the system itself with reality; and made us consider it something positive and non-hypothetical, when it is nothing other than a thought-image, a part of the mind.

This speculation seems nothing less than excessive when one takes account of the strange opinions put about in the scholarly world on the nature of our consciousness and faculty of knowing, how "the origin of our consciousness" and the possibility of explaining it through the action of the brain is disputed. Opinions and arguments whose absurdity and confused understanding strike us immediately if we only pay attention to the general foregoing reflections.

In fact we only know things of which we are conscious, but we infer the existence of unconscious things which are the cause our sensations.

It is these unconscious unknowns with which the natural sciences are principally concerned and to "explain" them is to forge links in the representation that we ourselves make of them. Even so science admits that what we perceive in a uniquely direct way, can also be perceived indirectly, that is to say through our senses, and this is perfectly understandable. If science didn't acknowledge that, its conceptual system would be incomplete. However, whether that system is susceptible to being augmented remains an open question. And when one considers what that would mean, the formation of an accurate mental image of what exists, indistinguishable *in any way* from reality, something which would in effect constitute the formation of a second reality in and by the first one, the answer here isn't difficult. There must necessarily be a difference, an awareness that the observing ego remains outside yet is itself an integral part of reality.

So we cannot draw conclusions from our mental representations of things which touch on the difference between them and external reality. We cannot represent our own ego to ourselves, just as we are unable to observe the back of our own eye. Science can form nothing more than an image, a σχημά[6], which corresponds to reality as a very ingenious robot does to a man. The persistent notions of man and the universe in the form of mechanical automatons is demonstration enough that we often speak of σχημά when we think we are speaking about reality.

These relatively simple reflections, but insufficiently taken into consideration, seem to us inescapable as soon as we become concerned with something intimately linked to that

---

[6] *Schematic representation.

part of a human being which is only perceptible in a direct manner.

The aversion of modern scholars to reflection and speculation in general is not inexplicable. No, not because it is difficult to think independently, but because we don't like to be deprived of the incontestable support of a widely recognised method. However, one cannot escape the fact that pure reflection is and remains the basis of all science and all methods, the source of the principles which guide our work, the supreme tribunal within whose jurisdiction lie the goal, the direction, the progress and the results. And the aversion must, above all, be overcome when dealing with those subjects which concern the mind and the self, or we will be exposed to the gravest of errors.

For example, it is an error to believe that psychology should attach itself directly to a science which follows a method characterised purely by proceeding from the known to the unknown. The "a priori" judgement that the mind's influence is limited to that which is perceptible through the indirect route, shows that we do believe this. Such a judgement is per se premature.

We scarcely discovered the phenomena of light and electricity by pure induction. Indeed we still have to deal with a great and imponderable unknown, notably whether the ether is continuous or not[7]. From that point to vital phenomena there is a still greater leap, so great that no one knows how to gauge it.

To make sense of living phenomena we have to reintroduce many unknown factors.

And the only sure way of getting there is the same as the one followed by the doctrine of evolution, which is to say assembling as many facts as possible without allowing *any* preconceived ideas to limit our conjecture. In other words, we have to accept with reservation, each fact such as it is and refrain from believing that we have the right to prejudge the issue.

With regard to psychological questions, nobody can sufficiently affirm this right. And whoever arrogates it to himself must be doing so on a more or less vague personal opinion based on such facts as he himself has brought together and observed. And the motives behind opposition to accepting the existence of inexplicable phenomena are invariably to do with sentiment, for example fear that the beauty or integrity of the scientific system will suffer, given

---

[7] The need for a material conception of ether led us to recognise a certain weight and a minimal resistance, however all empirical observations were in default of this idea.
"For the conveyance of radiation or light all ordinary matter is not only incompetent, but hopelessly and absurdly incompetent." (Prof. Oliver Lodge, The interstellar ether, *Fortnightly Review*, June 1893).

that the enemies of science and philosophy always follow faulty reasoning.

Let us cite a purely imaginary example: if someone notes the fact that an individual reacts contrary to the known rules of nutritive energy exchange put forward by Pettenkofer-Voit or Rubner, one couldn't say with scientific certainty that he must be mistaken because the law of conservation of energy renders such an anomaly impossible. If light and electricity cannot yet be completely transmuted into force and movement, how much more so vital processes. Who could deny with mathematical certainty the existence of forms of energy not — or only half — observed?

Now the laws of psychology and psycho-physiology are not laws, they are norms —things which have been regularly observed but do not yet have the constancy of the law of gravity. Is there a physiological observation which has been made more often than the temperature of the human body? And what physiological norm is as well established (by thousands of observations) as this one: the knowledge that the organism cannot survive a temperature higher than 44° or 45° centigrade? Yet a rigorous observation exists, leaving no doubt that a temperature of 50° persisted for several days in a patient who made a full recovery.[8]

It behoves us to follow here, as with all the sciences which have to deal with unknown factors, the same procedure which served Darwin in working out the laws of heredity; to gather together as many facts as possible and infer provisionally, without any preconceived conclusion and without the least inclination to doggedly maintain established hypotheses and conceptions.

This way of working is above all de rigueur when it comes to psychological questions where one has to deal with a factor which is not just unknown but essentially unknowable, which could never belong to the natural sciences because it cannot be admitted into the series of conceptions which form them, knowledge of the self, the observing ego.

It has been particularly difficult for doctors to maintain the aforesaid completely anti-dogmatic approach to vital phenomena, because urgent necessity and public impatience constrains them to implement each theoretical advance as soon as possible. Every new finding instantly becomes a basis for action.

---

[8] British Medical Journal 1875. Vol. I. p. 347. The Lancet 1875, Vol. I p.340. Cited by Dr. A. P. Mijers, Proceedings of the Society for Psychical Research. June 1893.

Pure scientific medicine is obliged to put into practice its discoveries — sometimes before they are conclusive — to deliver them into the hands of a crowd of practising doctors, anxious to extend the limits of their power over disease.

Each hypothesis prematurely affirmed in this way, becomes more or less public property and thus very quickly acquires a dogmatic cachet, which makes it all the more difficult to abandon at any given time. Is there any other science which has adopted such a large number of different systems, all put into practice, and all supplanted by their successor after heated debate? Even now, do we not see that it isn't *medical science* which reigns but rather one particular system: allopathic medicine, whose legitimacy is seriously contested by the claims of others, such as homeopathy or dosimetry.[9] Isn't this partly the fault of a power which is at the same time both spiritual and temporal? Far be it from us to wish to see another general system accredited. On the contrary we see in psychotherapy, systematically exercised, a correction of the cachet given to the reigning incomplete dogmatic principles, and above all a means of removing power from the enemies of science, whose principal weapon is without doubt

---

[9] * "Science of administering medicines in very small doses one after the other", propagated by Belgian doctor, Adolphe de Burggraeve.

"suggestion", and who exist only because physicians, far too riveted to their official system, don't understand suggestion and refuse to credit it.

What are the current principles, the views, which make it so difficult for modern medicine to accept the success of psychotherapy?

What conviction, what positive knowledge, what absolute truth is there in medicine or physiology, which refutes the disappearance of warts or luetic scotomas[10] or arthritis as a result of suggestion, backing up this denial with arbitrary statements such as: "this is a flagrant contradiction of all the laws of physiology."

It isn't easy to account for this. Conservation of energy has nothing to do with it. To claim that the effect of suggestion is impossible because it is a psychological phenomenon and the mind is necessarily powerless, is absurd and untenable.

Even if one goes along with this semblance of mindless automatism — necessitated by the nature of our knowledge — the whole world knows that purely psychological agents, that is to say those lending themselves only to direct personal observation, form *a part* of the apparently automatic chain. Conceptions, things which are only directly experienced, form essential links in the long chain which

---
[10] Blind spots caused by syphilis.

runs from sensation to action. Everybody knows this. There isn't any reason to regard these links as being of lesser importance, less active or of less powerful than other external indirect observables. One can accept as a rule, that the process unfolds with greater speed and energy when the pathway is shorter and the number of links less numerous, so that the addition of psychological factors slows down and obstructs the action, but there is no impossibility in principle.

One could say that the observation of the mind's extraordinary influence is all too rare. But that wouldn't get us anywhere. Physiology and pathology do not as a rule concern themselves with exceptionally rare facts, such as the very high temperature previously cited, splanchnic inversion, cancer cure, atavistic phenomena or anomalies in the growth and distribution of hair etc. etc., which nonetheless demand attention and serve to demonstrate that in biology we do not yet have laws but only more or less general norms.

Furthermore nobody has taken the trouble to research the phenomena which concern us here, they haven't been observed even when, so to speak, they imposed themselves, they have been overlooked and denied.

Indeed, although we are by no means ignorant of many of the objections raised, we are unaware of data sufficient to challenge the efficacy of suggestion in both functional and organic conditions. If one looks closely, in the end one only comes up with very vague personal statements such as: "all that seems very unbelievable"; "nobody really knows"; "that doesn't correlate with what we have known until now".

Now these dogmatic givens could only have arisen from the illusion that what has been known up till now corresponds perfectly with exact science. It isn't clear why an improvement in sclerotic plaques following the administration of silver nitrate should be held any more believable than one obtained through the use of suggestion.

Isn't it obvious that we are dealing here with vague impressions and opinions which give rise to the misconception that a concrete illness, observable by our senses, is more likely to be cured quickly by a concrete remedy; when one knows, when one is quite sure, that the mind is also involved in the curative process?

How could one forget it? Isn't this again a question of semi-conscious confusion of σχημά with reality, of the bodily machine which we perceive in our conceptual life through the medium of our senses, where we never detect — it goes without saying — any mental activity, with the living man of whose faculty of direct experiential observation we can persuade ourselves at every moment. But we aren't dealing with robots, we are dealing with living individuals to whom we are forced to accord a mind through the analogy of their functions with our own. We know that this mind also forms a link in the body's chain of organisation and that we are able to exercise an influence over it. What would be the principal objection?

It's an absolute illusion to think that current treatments rest on a more solid, scientific basis. That is quite impossible — even in the case of perfectly mechanical measures — because we have to interpose unknown factors in every curative process. Even the surgeon doesn't effect a cure without taking into account the bodily tissues' own functioning. The simplest medicines whose actions we know best, never take effect without the intermediary of our own plasma. We always have to introduce the idea of stimulus and response. What happens between the stimulus of living material and its consequent response is unknown.

The observed response is never determined theoretically but in an empirical manner. The intermediate links are incalculable. One can diminish the distance as much as possible, reduce to a minimum the transition between stimulus and response, but the closeness is only apparent, the crevasse remains just as large, since it continues to be the enormous crevasse between inductive and empirical knowledge, between a science proceeding unswervingly from the known to the unknown, and a science which dares not ever lose sight of the fact that an unknown factor exists, that it has covered up a gap, missed a link in the causal chain.

It is exactly this specious simultaneity, the apparent narrowness of the crevasse, which makes physicians act and think as if it didn't exist. Does the use of digitalis bear the mark of pure science? We study the action of alkaloids on the heart of a frog in the laboratory with the greatest exactitude and measurement. We learn to recognise the mechanism of action of the failing heart. Examination of the patient enables us to diagnose with phenomenal accuracy the different lesions, to detect immediately the symptoms of a default in compensation. Finally we know with almost mathematical precision how to administer the exact dose of the remedy at the desired time. But what happens between the moment when the liquid alkaloid moistens the ganglionic plasma and the moment when the cardiac fibres begin to contract with greater force, remains unknown. One talks of an "excitation" having been been transmitted. But how does that happen? We don't know the answer to that question. And thus the seeming exactitude and scientific precision of the remedy, disappears.

We can also transmit a stimulus, and cause one to be transmitted, by mental means. The mind exercises an influence over the structure and function of the tissues through the intermediary of the ganglionic plasma. This action of the plasma is the focus of all treatment. All therapeutic agents must cross this same bridge. So which among them follows a more scientific path?

Furthermore, one cannot deny that the role of the mind begins just where the action of other agents becomes problematic, that it forms the missing link in the known chain. So how is an "a priori" discussion of the limits of its action possible? What attitude is more befitting than to wait and carefully observe the facts?

It goes without saying that the limit of all therapeutic action is set by this same function of the plasma. One can help the action of the tissues, one cannot either replace or increase it. This applies however to *all* medicines, mental or otherwise, since none can act other than through this means. Nothing is stranger than the scornful remark, raised as an objection, that the mind cannot restore parts of the body which have been destroyed. Is there indeed any medicine that has this power?

The doctor can do no more than come to the aid of the organism's own healing capacity. He does it with treatments, psychological or otherwise. If the point of intervention differs the point of application remains the same. In the final analysis the mode of action comes back to the same thing in both cases. Mental agents act from the centre to the periphery, others proceed from the periphery to the centre. Experience alone must decide which is better. To begin with, one is no more important than the other.

And if one of them were to be less important than the other, it is certainly not psychotherapy. Saying that isn't seeking to overstate its power. Clearly in many cases this power is insufficient. Strong medicines and direct action often have an infinitely more effective influence, above all on the coarser subordinate parts of the organism, over which the mind can only act with difficulty, encountering inevitable constraints. But, as we have already remarked, all things being equal, psychotherapy wins due to its purer and more natural principle. It helps the organism to cure itself; it is less foreign, abnormal and debilitating than other treatment modalities. Its mode of action proceeds from the centre to the periphery without having to weaken the organism with all kinds of external support. It tends to consolidate. Applied with discernment, with the reinforcement of the conscious will wedded to a methodical longterm practice, it reawakens the body's force of resistance, it conserves and augments this precious force thanks to which the tissues and the whole organism react against deleterious influences and repair themselves. It would scarcely serve us, it might even cause serious damage, to refuse from outraged faithfulness to theoretical principles to recognise this force as a special one and to give it a name.

Let us suppose it proven that the consideration we put forward earlier is invalid, that a mind does not include a subjective self and that the representation of this self is not an impossibility. Let us further suppose that we can form such a complete conception of a man that the idea itself has a mind, that is to say that one can see in this representation how man observes himself. On considering this possibility, nobody could deny that we haven't yet worked this miracle and that we are not even close to doing so.

For as long as we are unable to represent our own mind, that is to say we conceive of it in currently known forms, but we continue to notice that living things differ from dead ones in so far as they possess a certain functional subjectivity; indicating the presence of a more or less primitive form of self-awareness; for so long we think, there isn't the least harm in speaking for practical purposes of a vital force or vital energy.

And indeed these expressions are still used in the doctrine of heredity concerning correlative and alternating variations. Darwin employs the word "vital power" when he speaks of the relative quantity of energy at the disposal of the organism for growth, for the power of resistance and for regeneration[11].

It is an entity, a well defined conception. Organs require a good deal of vital energy in order to develop and they become extinct unless there are exceptionally serious forces opposed to this outcome. The idea that the force expended in growth or regeneration is subtracted from the total amount of available energy at the cost of the force of resistance, derives from this rule.

This same idea also occurs in the chapter on degeneration and extinction of races as a result of constant external conditions. It is of little matter whether one day we will be able to bring this energy into line with other known forms of energy. For the time being the connection between them is absolutely obscure and under these conditions, judged from the purely practical point of view, the word is perfectly entitled to exist.

---

[11] *Descent of man.* Ed. 1888. P. 503.

How many similar expressions are we not aware of in medicine which have been in use for a long time and still not disappeared; they couldn't, above all because medicine is a practical science. What does the word "tone' signify? Why do we call some medicines "fortifying"? What does the word "asthenia" mean? What does one mean by "fortify" when one prescribes fortifying drugs?

These expressions and many others still very much in use in practice all relate to more or less clear hypotheses concerning particular symptoms. Does a consumptive's appetite increase, does he feel more refreshed, less fatigued, and can he allow himself more exercise after taking a lot of albumin or a decoction of quinine, so that we say we've given him tone, that the tonic has fortified him? But whether something happens in his organism, corresponding to a mechanical or physical increase in tone is clearly indemonstrable. And what force we have added, what latent energies or powers we have augmented, in what way we have, so to speak, fortified him, is completely nebulous.

We have temporarily, directly or indirectly, augmented nutritive exchanges, combustion, and we have perhaps stimulated some tissues — and consequently the patient may present certain objective and subjective signs of improvement. These are real facts. The terms used to describe them are dependant on vague more or less personal hypotheses. Wouldn't it be just as scientific and correct, perhaps more so, to speak here of having awoken vital energy? Just as scientific because the term "vital force" indicates a group defined by phenomena which we haven't succeeded in analysing. While other terms more or less imply that we have made a successful analysis. They suggest more than they can justify, and the more general term isn't flawed with that excess.

Clearly that is of no secondary importance. Agreed generality presents more security than dubious precision. It is dangerous to think that one knows what one is doing when it is not really the case. This danger manifests itself particularly here. We have abandoned a very useful general conception in favour of following an inclination for precision, and none of the remaining terms has been able to replace it.

Why not? Vital energy signifies a definite enduring entity, linked to a particular organism. A collection of forces so perfectly connected that they form throughout life a single persistent thing[12], just as long as the organism continues to exist. Now that isn't conveyed by any of the less general

---

[12] No, "immutable".

terms, nevertheless herein resides an eminent practical danger.

If one considers the organism as if it were a stove that one only has to light or a machine that only has to be filled with fuel or again a robot which has to be reassembled, one is soon led to believe that one has done enough in providing the necessary fuel, repairing the apparent damage and preventing it from wearing out as much as possible. But in this way of thinking one has forgotten to take account of the growth and regenerative force which is intimately involved in the force of total resistance. A force evidently dependant on heredity, whose rules are still mysterious and insufficiently understood. A force whose potential size seems determined from birth and which cannot be increased but is at most retained at its original level. Thus it is susceptible to stimulation but not amplification, so that it constitutes, so to speak, a provision which one has to use economically. It is a force which can exhaust itself in an alternating or vicarious manner, to the extent that it benefits certain parts or specific periods of life at the expense of other parts, or to the detriment of the whole of later existence.

This is a type of exhaustion not in anyway comparable to the deterioration of a machine which wears out. Local deterioration has no influence over the rest of the machine's construction. It isn't possible to stimulate a machine in such way that the worn out part continues to temporarily fulfil its functions only to subsequently provoke more rapid ruin of the total structure.

A machine does not keep in reserve a stock of resistive or restorative power, proceeds which it can enjoy but which it can also consume. What happens in an organism can sometimes be compared to the aforesaid destruction (diminution in vascular elasticity, functional neuroses and atrophies etc.). But something else is also produced, something of a much more complicated nature to which the application of the machine analogy would be impossible and dangerous. What machine possesses, as our organs do, parts which gain in force and strength through use? In what machine does action at the same time constitute a stimulation? What machine reacts against noxious influences by building, up to a certain limit, its force of resistance?

In what machine does the remarkable reigning principle exist, belonging to all living organisms, of a constant level of functioning, below which all noxious influences and also all the work done are profitable to the economy, while only above and beyond does the damage and the loss begin? That muscle grows and strengthens itself to a certain point through use, atrophying and becoming paralysed as a result of overwork, evidences this principle.

In a machine, all damage is directly disadvantageous, all use brings with it wear and tear, all work done constitutes an immediate loss, only remedied by refuelling. If one wished to treat the human organism according to these principles, one would believe it best to avoid all challenging influences, relieving man of all work and simply supplying him with more fuel, that is to say food, when the ability to work threatens to disappear.

If the application of such a system can preserve a machine, it can destroy an organism. Too little external resistance is as detrimental as too much. Lack of action gives rise to a state of decline in every part of the organism, a state of decline and weakness for which there is no analogy in the stiffness of an idle machine. Here it's rust or something similar, a consequence of external noxious influences. For the organism, the absence of these noxious influences constitutes precisely the damage. Too much protection is weakening.

Everybody also knows that one cannot arbitrarily compensate all energy loss with a food supplement. It is true that when everything is functioning well within certain limits, there is an equivalence between work done and food intake. But from the moment that normal function is disturbed or as soon as the organism finds itself overworked, one can't compensate for the defect with extra food.

In the most well nourished organism, one can find atrophies caused by disuse just as often as overuse. That proves that the vital economy isn't as simple as some would wish to purport, since neediness wouldn't occur in the midst of excessive abundance. An input matching the output would be the ideal situation.

We tend to exceed this measure. Under those conditions things become dysfunctional, there's no point in blindly increasing the input of food, as is so often done in practice. In such a case food no longer simply serves to cover the expended energy, but it acts as a stimulus, and the surplus must be digested and eliminated to the detriment of the organism.

There is nothing so dangerous in medical practice as oversimple interpretations. One could compare the increase in volume of muscle under the mechanical influence of afferent vessels to the auto-regulation of some machines. But how to explain the weakening of the optic nerve when deprived of its stimulus, light, if not by lack of attentive effort? Indeed in strabismus,[13] isn't the retina rendered particularly insensitive by lack of stimulus from the unknown central action which determines attention?

This fact and yet others lead us to suppose that auto-regulation of muscle is not simply a mechanical process, but has a more complicated character.

In the final analysis the organism possesses the functions of protection and defence. On might almost say that the total structure is formed with the aim of protecting the whole. The skin reacting to variations in temperature is the most salient example. And everybody also knows that the same skin reaction constitutes a stimulus for the protective faculty, in so far as inaction weakens this function due to lack of stimulation. Skin which hasn't been exposed to changes in temperature for a long time, loses its ability to act and its reactions are diminished.

Now this altogether special property of vital functions, belonging uniquely to living phenomena, and which machines are not gifted with, leads to the therapeutic conceptions *of exercise* and *hardening* with far reaching practical consequences. Exercise is the improvement obtained by the stimulus of action, hardening is the same idea applied to the protective functions, thus the exercise of

---

[13] * Squint.

the power of resistance. In both cases we have to be aware that there is a limit beyond which direct damage will quickly occur. And one of the most important subjects of hygiene should be the exact study of the level of these limits.

Medicine has occupied itself too little with all of this up till now, because it thinks it has to follow an inductive course and because it forgets that it works practically all the time at the heights where all induction abandons us and where empiricism and deduction must be our principal guides; because it illicitly cultivates from preference branches of its sphere of practical activity which are closest neighbours to exact science.

Wishing to follow the theories and materialist technologies of exact science which are perfectly licit, in an absolutely illicit way, it has come to consider man as a machine or robot and to treat him as such.

It neglects the important notion of vitality, and thus continually loses sight of the unique principles covered by this concept, although they are generally known. It does this by unjustifiably extending the theories and hypotheses permitted in exact science to its sphere of active action.

It is true that one finds an exposition of these principles in manuals treating pathology and therapeutics[14]; however they

---

[14] See e.g. F.R. Hoffman, Vorlesungen über Allgemeine Therapie.

are not accorded due attention and application. Only an insignificant part of the time devoted to the study of medicine is allocated to the deep exploration of these issues, which from a practical point of view are of greater interest and should form the quintessence of medicine properly so called.

And if the faculty were to condescend to make a practical scientific study of the systems belonging to charlatans and laymen, the most renowned of which seriously undermine its prestige through their amazing success, it would nearly always find these factors that it has been so wrong to ignore: exercise, hardening and suggestion.

All these systems and so to speak, natural medical methods, derive in effect from one idea: vitality, an idea abandoned too early by medicine, or rather they put to use the power of the mind of which science guided by superficial theoretical considerations hasn't taken sufficient account.

Psycho-therapy in the widest sense comprises the corrective for these faults.

Psycho-therapy thus redirects the misfocused attention of doctors to these important phenomena which represent the idea of vitality. The power of the body to protect and regenerate itself. And then the role that the mind plays in this.

It insists on a more precise study of the nature of this vitality and its mental action. It insists on the questions: What determines the magnitude of this vitality? How can it be preserved? What stimulates it? What releases it? What is the nature of these stimulants? How does a transient stimulus give rise to a long lasting degree of exhaustion? What is the normal and desired stimulus? What are the levels of limit where benefit changes to disadvantage?

Again, it insists on studying how best one can activate the mental stimulus, implying that this is the normal stimulus. It studies the extent of this action and how it can be controlled. It seeks to identify appropriate cases where it is very desirable to replace abnormal external stimuli e.g. chemical, electrical or mechanical treatments, with mental stimuli.

Since we have neglected vitality, it would appear that doctors have no other aim than to procure a state of well-being and a semblance of health for their patients in the shortest possible time, as if this end sanctified all the means. One goes on stimulating and fortifying without worrying about the nature and consequences of those stimuli. One prescribes iron, arsenic, strychnine, potassium iodide and numerous other medicines over months and years, and the only thing which guides the doctor is the transient increase in wellbeing. The empirical deduction there is the occasional observation of such an increase, the inductive theory is a consideration of the chemical action of these agents.

Nobody is interested in or has collected data on the extent to which vitality, the power of resistance and regeneration, is undermined by his therapy.

Basing oneself on the "scientific" mechanical theory, one continues to blindly feed patients, without taking account of whether in effect one is removing a stimulus and thus inadvertently exhausting them. One protects individuals in all sorts of ways, without worrying whether this protection in fact constitutes a permanent advantage for the organism. One does this in order to avoid and rule out all noxious influences, through the use of all sorts of treatments aimed at momentary benefit, without wondering whether in doing so one removes one of the essential conditions of life, as much for the individual as for the whole race.

The narrowness of this approach doesn't sit well with a science so highly thought of. It's not impossible that one day the degeneration of the race will be attributed, and with good cause, to this narrowness. Practical medicine pays too much attention to the individual, where it should be concerned with the whole race. It pursues a system of mending and patching, in line with the fleeting wishes of the individual, where it ought to be acting forcefully according to those principles and ideas which the extended study of vital phenomena gives to the needs and necessities of all humanity. The doctor is still too much of a barber.

And the practical application of the principles of psychotherapy will without doubt be thwarted by the apparently piffling difficulty, but actually eminently powerful one, of knowing that the doctor finds himself obliged to prescribe something at each visit or each consultation.

How many soporifics, narcotics, analgesics and tranquillisers does one prescribe for instance, out of blind compassion, in order to procure transient relief, without possessing any scientific conviction that one is acting in the long term interests of the patient? The doctor must have the courage to know how to refuse to suppress the pain and insomnia of patients when he is scientifically convinced that it is in their best interest. Just as the fear which an operation inspires in a patient doesn't affect the surgical treatment.

We have taught a good number of our patients to bear their afflictions without ceaselessly searching for new palliatives. And we have frequently seen that the too long neglected power of the body to regenerate asserted itself, and that an equilibrium was spontaneously restored from the moment that the medication which had been taken for years was withdrawn and thus ceased to oppose this restoration.

There is no need to point out once again the manic surgical interventions advocated in chronic neuroses (above all the outrageous tendency to oophorectomy) and the desire which haunts almost all nerve patients to submit themselves to a gynaecological treatment. The reaction is clearly already beginning to show itself; it is beyond doubt that the honour of having widely contributed to this turnaround of opinion comes down to suggestion.

But these errors are also based on the same false idea that all therapy must find its point of application outside the self. They are the inevitable consequence of the external and palliative nature of our treatments.

Above all current medical science has a need for a fundamental study of vitality, of the power of resistance, of personal defence and regeneration. The laboratory alone is insufficient for this purpose, a critical examination of a large collection of facts is necessary, along lines which led to the development of the doctrine of evolution.

The importance of taking account of this force in our cultivated society must seem evident to everybody. Do we not see that this force is all the greater the lower we descend in the animal series? Do we not see that the regeneration of damaged tissue, even complicated whole organs (such as the tail, the foot, the eye) are still produced in the ranks of the vertebrates? To these facts must be added the observation that the force of regeneration is greater in uncivilised people than in the most civilised, e.g. perforating wounds of the abdomen, absolutely mortal in the European, heal perfectly well in the Negro, conditions of hygiene and good care being equal in both cases.

And isn't it all the more striking, that medicine, instead of harnessing this precious force to oppose debilitation, has in effect done nothing other than promote this weakening through its palliative system.

It goes without saying that the corrective of psycho-therapeutic success will only exercise its practical influence on general therapeutics very slowly and gradually. Only little by little will irrational overprescribing of medicines disappear and the ideas of exercise, hardening and suggestion become accepted. Just as phlebotomy, the prescription of simples and that of excessive pharmaceutical recipes, have gradually been put out of use.

Provisionally, a systematic application of psycho-therapy will not be able to be carried out by the general practitioner.

It is not only impossible to break with a custom from the outset, but the defiance of the patient, the fear of "hypnotism", the lack of experience and confidence, the time involved, the difficulty and the moral courage that the application demands, will present insurmountable problems for the general practitioner who is intent on following the principle.

The current resistance is so great, that every unfavourable turn in the course of an illness will, almost inevitably, be put down to the unusual treatment. One cannot defy all this in specialist practice. Even we have to refrain from treating patients presenting the initial signs of severe mental illness. Although there may be good reason to think we could produce an improvement in the illness or slow it down, we can be sure that the first manifestation of a manic state would be attributed to "hypnotism", and that this incident wouldn't fail to feed the prejudices concerning the awful dangers of suggestion for a long time.

For the time being one cannot successfully apply psycho-therapy with the necessary rigour, other than in a hospital, a sanatorium, a clinic or a specialist practice.

There one can set out the rules to which whomsoever wishes to be treated has to submit his will; there one finds a leading example, the calming and suggestive influence of a milieu where several other patients are being treated in the same way. There one can give the necessary time and personal attention to each patient. In certain cases, in order to be assured of success, one must — as is now generally recognised — call upon isolation, a severe regime and assiduous surveillance. Now these psychological resources can just about only be found in a sanatorium or specialist clinic.

The results that we are publishing here do not claim to present all the details with the precision that one is accustomed to finding in the work of academic researchers who have at their disposal everything they need for their research. We are simply presenting what we have been able to gather together, guaranteeing the distinctive character of the facts we put before you. Their interpretation is only provisional. These are only pointers capable of serving a more thorough and fundamental enquiry by those more competent than ourselves. We do consider however that here, where we are dealing with a science which is still in its infancy, all these pointers and provisional results will be of use.

# GENERAL SUMMARY

## OF THE

**Statistics 1889 — 1893**

*Covering all cases treated between 5 May 1887 and 30 June 1893*
## A. Diseases of the nervous system.

| | I Organic conditions | II Grand neuroses/ Hysterical conditions | III Mental illnesses | IV Neuropathic conditions | V Neuralgias, pains |
|---|---|---|---|---|---|
| **No/sex of patients entering service.** | | | | | |
| Men | 36 | 120 | 67 | 151 | 5 |
| Women | 27 | 203 | 55 | 96 | 11 |
| **Total** | 63 | 323 | 122 | 247 | 16 |
| **Degree of hypnotic influence.** | | | | | |
| a. Refractory. | 3 | 18 | 12 | 15 | 7 |
| b. Light sleep. | 21 | 119 | 70 | 123 | 91 |
| c. Deep sleep. | 25 (sic) ? 35 | 132 | 36 | 85 | 51 |
| d. Somnambulism | 4 | 54 | 4 | 24 | 17 |
| **Total** | 63 (sic) | 323 | 122 | 247 | 166 |
| **Age in years.** | | | | | |
| a. 1 - 10. | 4 | 7 | 0 | 19 | 2 |
| b. 11 - 20 | 4 | 40 | 7 | 58 | 19 |
| c. 21 - 40 | 25 | 215 | 70 | 104 | 79 |
| d. 41 - 60 | 18 | 52 | 38 | 52 | 56 |
| e. 61 - 80 | 12 | 9 | 7 | 14 | 10 |
| **Total** | 63 | 323 | 122 | 247 | 166 |
| **Results of treatment.** | | | | | |
| a. No effect. | 19 | 55 | 30 | 36 | 25 |
| b. Slight improvement. | 21 | 59 | 23 | 55 | 33 |
| c. Marked improvement. | 12 | 100 | 25 | 50 | 23 |
| Cure. | 1 | 91 | 25 | 77 | 58 |
| Unknown. | 10 | 18 | 19 | 29 | 15 |
| **Total** | 63 | 323 | 122 | 247 | 166 |

*Covering all cases treated between 5 May 1887 and 30 June 1893*
## B. Diseases of diverse organs or systems (not nervous system).

| | VI Functional troubles linked with Internal diseases | VII Functional troubles linked with External diseases | VIII Fevers | IX Chlorosis Menstrual problems | X Surgical anaesthesia | Totals | Proportion |
|---|---|---|---|---|---|---|---|
| No/sex of patients | | | | | | | |
| Men | 63 | 21 | 0 | 0 | 1 | 529 | 48.57% |
| Women | 44 | 15 | 1 | 16 | 7 | 560 | 51.42 |
| Total | 107 | 36 | 1 | 16 | 8 | 1089 | |
| Degree of hypnotic influence. | | | | | | | |
| a. Refractory. | 0 | 2 | 0 | 0 | 1 | 58 | 5.33% |
| b. Light sleep. | 23 | 13 | 1 | 5 | 0 | 406 | 42.78 |
| c. Deep sleep. | 77 | 20 | 0 | 6 | 3 | 445 | 40.87 |
| d. Somnambulism | 7 | 1 | 0 | 5 | 4 | 120 | 11.61 |
| Total | 107 | 36 | 1 | 16 | 8 | 1089 | |
| Age in years. | | | | | | | |
| a. 1 - 10. | 0 | 3 | 0 | 0 | 0 | 35 | |
| b. 11 - 20 | 23 | 2 | 0 | 3 | 1 | 136 | |
| c. 21 - 40 | 77 | 23 | 0 | 9 | 6 | 567 | |
| d. 41 - 60 | 77 | 6 | 1 | 4 | 1 | 281 | |
| e. 61 - 80 | 7 | 2 | 0 | 0 | 0 | 70 | |
| Total | 107 | 36 | 1 | 16 | 8 | 1089 | |
| Results of treatment. | | | | | | | |
| a. No effect. | 16 | 11 | 1 | 1 | 0 | 194 | 17.81% |
| b. Slight improvement. | 31 | 6 | 0 | 1 | 0 | 229 | 21.02 |
| c. Marked improvement. | 23 | 9 | 0 | 2 | 2* | 258 | 23.00 |
| Cure. | 32 | 7 | 0 | 11 | 6** | 308 | 28.28 |
| Unknown. | 5 | 3 | 0 | 1 | 0 | 100 | 9.18 |
| Total | 107 | 36 | 1 | 247 | 8 | 1089 | |

*Incomplete anaesthesia    **Complete Anaesthesia

# CLINICAL OBSERVATIONS

# A. GROUP I
## Organic affections of the Nervous System

The number of patients belonging to this group is relatively small because current opinion, above all that of doctors, excludes *a priori*[15] improvement brought about by psychological means. For this reason such patients have exceptional recourse to us and only the most serious cases are referred when all other treatments have been exhausted.

In spite of that we are happy to have been able to improve, and do some good, in the majority of cases presenting. In those completely refractory to our psychological means, all other treatment modalities had proved or subsequently proved to be equally useless.

We conclude from this fact that in curable cases, the cure or improvement can be obtained just as well through psychological means as through other methods. Only further research can decide the question: whether the different approaches offer equal chances of cure or not?

We understand that to study the question in depth, one would also have to apply psycho-therapy to early onset cases of illness.

---
[15] * In principle.

It goes without saying that we have no intention of definitively proscribing medicines in use until now, notably the so-called specifics; we understand the need for their prescription if the state of the illness demands it or if psycho-therapy alone remains unable to meet the need. However to fail to make use of psychological means other than in the last analysis, only when all other forms of treatment have been exhausted, seems to us a bad tactic. On the contrary, we think it is far more rational to ascertain as a first step what can be obtained through the *vis medicatrix naturae*[16] and from a psychological stimulus, and to turn to other more abnormal and violent *stimuli* only as a last resort.

**OBS. 1**

SYPHILITIC HEMIPLEGIA & EPILEPSY; MIXED TREATMENT, SMALL IMPROVEMENT.

A captain in the army of the Dutch-Indies, aged 37 years, requested my care on the 29 April 1892.

In 1880 he had contracted an indurated chancre followed by an exanthema which was treated with mercurial rubs. In 1882 specific iritis.

In January 1891, several months after his wedding, he was struck by a paralysis of his left side. Treatment with sublimate injections[17]

---

[16] * The healing power of nature.

[17] * Mercuric chloride.

and high doses of potassium iodide. Partial improvement. Temporary sick leave. Repatriated, the patient was treated with anti-luetics[18], massage and electricity in the Amsterdam Military and Nymège hospitals. From the latter hospital he was referred to me.

*Present state.* Small, strong man, very muscular, irritable temperament. Paralysis of the left facial nerve; fixed stare caused by synechiae[19]. These disabilities and frequent bursts of inappropriate laughter give him a more or less fatuous physiognomy. A minor speech impediment which the patient claims to have had since infancy.

The left arm is partially contracted, the left leg is paralysed and contracted. Cutaneous and tendinous reflexes are exaggerated on the left side. When walking the patient stamps on his left heel and flexes his leg imperfectly, he holds his elbow out, the left forearm is pronated and the finger contracted. He cannot lift his hand higher than his nose. Sleep, digestion and stools are unremarkable.

From the 29 April to the 11th of the following August I treated the patient with suggestion and systematic exercise of the affected limbs, both during and outside the hypnotic state, and total abstinence from medication.

The patient's state gradually improved. On the 10 August I noted: The patient can grasp a glass or cup with his left hand, bring it to his mouth and drink without spilling a drop, he can use a hammer

---

[18] *Anti-syphilitic drugs.

[19] *Adhesion of the iris to cornea or lens.

and nails. These movements are always exercised clumsily. It is to be noted that in the past the patient was ambidextrous. When playing cards, it is now possible for him to hold his hand on the left side which he previously couldn't succeed in doing. He walks better, no longer needs to lean on his wife's arm. He climbs and descends stairs at a gradient of twenty degrees with his arms folded behind his back. When walking he completely flexes his leg, however the flexion is too slow and the extension is too forceful; a transient tremor of the limb can be observed after this movement. He places his foot much more flatly on the ground, he walks less on his heel. He still holds his elbow out. Can describe a semi-circle with his left arm in the horizontal plane, can bring his hand to the middle of his head and to his occiput and extend his fingers. However his limb quickly becomes tired and he needs a rest of several minutes before these movements can be repeated. If the exercise is repeated more than twice in a row, his arm begins to tremble and his nervous laugh begins. His general state is excellent. Large sexual appetite.

The following day while walking with his wife the patient suddenly stopped in his tracks, closed his eyes and lost consciousness for one or two seconds; he didn't fall, the fingers on his left hand were violently contracted. He came back and lay down on his bed, after which he notified me. I found him perfectly calm, however during my examination his eyes stared vacantly, his face became congested, both his arms stiffened and crossed spasmodically over his chest and he lost consciousness. The fit lasted less than a minute. A mercurial and iodide treatment was immediately instituted.

The epileptic fits grew in number and duration over the following three days, then they began to diminish and ceased completely on the tenth day.

I assured myself that this series of epileptic fits hadn't resulted in any loss to the patient of the advantages obtained from suggestive therapy. He left our clinic on the following 29 August.

We would have wished to have been able to treat a greater number of visual disturbances. The classic observations of Professor Delboeuf in Liège[20], all sorts of gossip and old wives tales of miraculous cures of blindness, and again the success of many charlatans, leads us to believe that suggestion has a role to play in ophthalmology. Our personal setbacks in several cases proves little; only a large number of trials and observations could prove the point.

In 1889 one of us presented a clear cut case of tabes dorsalis to the Amsterdam Medical Association in which excruciating pains had totally disappeared as the result of suggestion, while the ataxia improved so much that Romberg's sign[21] was abolished and the patient's gait

---

[20] On the extent of the curative action of hypnotism. Hypnotism applied to conditions of the visual organ, by Professor J. Delboeuf with the collaboration of Professor Nuel and Doctor Leplat. — Paris 1890. Felix Alcan.

[21] *Loss of postural control when eyes closed.

became steadier. That improvement has been maintained to the present time. This is one of our most successful cases. In other cases of ataxia we have only been able to obtain a diminution in pain or transient amelioration of variable duration, while failing to secure a lasting halt to the course of the illness. The transient effect of suggestion in these cases is clearly apparent and excludes beyond all doubt fortuitous coincidence.

Some of the most distinguished authors have also noted the favourable effect of suggestion in cases of locomotor ataxia. See among others: Bernheim[22], Bérillon[23], Wetterstrand[24]. The following observation shows for a fact the termination of a non-functional[25] pathological process by mean of suggestion.

---

[22] Etudes nouvelles 1891. Octave Doin. Paris

[23] Revue de l'hypnotisme 1892

[24] Der Hypnoyismus und seine Anwendung in der parkt. Medizin. 1891.

[25] *Organic.

## OBS. 2

TRANSVERSE MYELITIS[26](?) COMPLICATED BY HYSTERIA; MARKED IMPROVEMENT

Mrs X X, born 1852, married 1870, is the mother of ten healthy children. No family history. In 1874 she fell out of a hammock on to her coccyx.

Following the advice of her doctor, she stayed in bed for several months or at least maintained a lying position, and in addition she wore a steel corset to relieve the weight of her upper trunk on her vertebral column. Four years later she experienced serious family grief. The present illness only started in 1883, with pains in her right big toe. At first she paid little attention, however the pains increased and gradually began to affect her when walking uphill.

She presented to me on 14 January 1890 complaining of continuous pain of a nervous character in her left hip and intermittent pains in parts of her back, chest and side; above all she often felt pain between her shoulder-blades. There was a paresis of the right lower limb.

The patient was also troubled by a persistent cough and light bad sleep; she didn't normally sleep for more than two hours at a time. On waking, an anxious sensation, as if she had done something wrong. She appears scatty, quickly forgets things and has little nervous crises from time to time accompanied by tears which relieve her.

---

[26] * Inflamation of the spinal cord.

Mrs X X often suffers from tic douloureux. During the course of her illness difficulties in speech and right arm movements occurred. She had paraesthesiae in her right leg (feelings of contusion, and doughiness).

The patient seemed healthy, she was well nourished, a little on the chubby side. Varices in the legs since her most recent pregnancies. The lower right limb was weak. The least exercise caused tonic and clonic spasms mainly in the extensor muscles of the big toe. The same phenomenon also occurred in her left limb but to a lesser degree.

Sensitivity in her right lower limb was slightly blunted. Her cutaneous reflexes were accentuated, the patellar reflex was normal. On the right, the Achilles tendon reflex was absent. Paresis of the calf. Paralysis of the anterior tibial muscle. The femoral triceps and right anterior were weakened. The right lower leg measured at its greatest thickness was one centimetre less than the left, an effect due to atrophy of the anterior tibial muscle.

The reaction to electrical stimulus of the perineal nerve was perfectly normal; there was total abolition of galvanic and faradic contractility in the anterior tibial muscle; no degenerative reaction.

Examination of internal genital organs gave negative results, other than some exaggerated sensitivity to pressure in the region of the great ischiatic notch.

Anaesthesia of the anus and occasional involuntary bowel evacuation.

Nothing abnormal in thoracic or abdominal organs. The phenomena presented by her arms and hands are of a subjective order. There are no tremors, nystagmus or contractures; there are no symptoms of sciatica.

She experiences a sensation of laxity as if prolapse were about to occur in her genital organs. Urine examination gives a specific gravity of 1.013 and shows an absence of sugar, indica, and bile pigments. There are traces of albumin and many vaginal and bladder epithelial cells

The spinal apophysis of the eighth dorsal vertebra is prominent and very sensitive to pressure.

Although there isn't the least doubt that hysterical symptoms complicate the illness syndrome, the presence of organic problems in the spinal cord is more than likely, notably chronic degeneration of the grey matter of the nerve roots in the lumbar region: a transverse or ascending myelitis. The trauma which preceded the illness, the observed prominence and deviation of the eighth thoracic vertebra with hyperaesthesia, the atrophy, the paralysis, and the absence of reaction to electrical stimulation of the tibialis anterior, the lack of tendon reflexes, the anaesthesia in the anal region and the continuous localised sensitivity reactions, all point toward the diagnosis of an organic nervous condition.

The hysterical phenomena are more or less confined to bursts of tears or mad laughter, insomnia, and to a certain degree, jitteriness. Paresis, contractures, cramps and localised loss of sensation have never been observed other than in the regions mentioned where they have been present for years.

The authorities previously consulted prescribed: absolute bedrest, no exercise, avoid all attempts at walking; hot needles in the back, bandaging with tincture of iodine. Potassium iodide ( 1.5 to 3 grams b.d.), silver nitrate (30 to 40 mg. b.d.) and sodium bromide in high doses, to be taken orally. Hypodermic injections of strychnine; electricity; a season of baths at Nauheim.

A large part of this programme had been carried out. The patient had kept to a regime of absolute rest for a year, without gaining the least benefit; on the contrary her pains were aggravated and the difficulty in walking had increased.

So she was referred to me. I advised abandoning the whole programme and from then on all medication both internal and external was stopped, psycho-therapy being the sole treatment.

Bedrest was replaced with other activities and moderate exercise.

From the first session I succeeded in putting the patient into a light sleep. Her awakening was obtained by a small sign or else she woke up spontaneously when she calculated that I wanted her to come round. Her capacity for observation sharpened during the sleep in a remarkable way. For example she came round almost punctually following an order given 12, 15, 25 minutes or an hour and a half beforehand, without ever being out by more than a minute.

Throughout the duration of the treatment the depth of sleep elicited in my patient scarcely altered; on rare occasions her drowsiness was disturbed, sometimes as the result of some kind of agitation, so that the hypnosis became lighter and I could hardly maintain her sleeping state.

To begin with I contented myself with treatment aimed at improving her general condition, calming and relieving pain and improving her nocturnal sleep. Once that effect had been obtained, I proceeded to make her do systematic exercises of the affected limb during hypnotic sleep. I succeeded admirably; after a few sessions the patient could stand up on the paralysed leg, she lifted her knee quite well when walking. However the anterior tibial muscle continued and still continues to malfunction. There remains a tendency for her to walk on the external edge of her foot and it is impossible for her to place it flat on the ground, it always turns outward. Also the patient drags her foot while walking. Despite this I noted on the 28 January 1890 that she permitted herself a walk for half an hour, the pains and the cramps had diminished; she slept perfectly well at night even though I had discontinued the potassium bromide which she used to take regularly.

All exercise was painful during the first few minutes, however this gradually improved. During the summer of 1890 the patient was already walking for two hours and more.

Today, that is to say three and a half years after the beginning of the treatment, Mrs X X continues to benefit from the improvement obtained. However, to achieve this result, frequently repeated suggestions and incessant care are necessary. The patient, naturally active and busy, is inclined to overwork. The inevitable consequences are first insomnia, then an exacerbation of pains in the back and hip, the reappearance of cramps, difficulty in walking, general malaise and finally melancholia. She remembered the negative prognosis that the doctors caring for her before me had given, and she despairs of a cure. Everything begins again. The worry and anxiety has to be combatted by a prolonged hypnotic sleep (of 2 to 3 hours) and by forceful suggestions reassuring her of a good night's sleep and the disappearance of her pains and motor troubles. Her equilibrium is only maintained thanks to a calm life, with much rest alternating with regular moderate exercise. Her emotional states are also causes of occasional aggravation and necessitate intervention with appropriate suggestions. Concomitant symptoms such as nervous cough, tic douloureux etc are easily overcome by suggestion.

On one occasion I extracted two molars during a hypnotic sleep without any notable suffering on the part of the patient; she felt the operation happening, but didn't suffer any severe pain.

Today, after three and a half years the advantages obtained persist. The atrophy and the paresis have not increased. The overall direction is always towards progress, the pains occur rarely and then only at times when she is very tired.

We are very much aware that multiple sclerosis although falling into the category of incurable illness, can present periods of recovery and remission of symptoms.

Any treatment producing a notable remission would without doubt be highly suspect to everybody. Now we believe that in the following observation suggestion has fulfilled this role in such a clear cut way that it cannot be ignored. The improvement wasn't merely obtained *post* but without doubt *propter suggestionem*.[27]

Bernheim in his *Etudes nouvelles* describes a case of multiple sclerosis in which the tremor and the titubation disappeared as a result of several sessions of hypnotic suggestion.

Fontan and Ségard (*Eléments de médecine suggestive*) similarly obtained a marked improvement of all symptoms in a case of chronic diffuse myelitis (a mild form of multiple sclerosis).

## OBS. 3.

MULTIPLE SCLEROSIS; SMALL IMPROVEMENT.

On the 27 June 1890 a young woman aged 27, dressmaker, was brought to see me by her parents. She had had to give up her work long before then. The doctor who was looking after her had requested urgent treatment in a hospital, however neither the patient nor her parents took to this advice. She had had difficulty in swallowing for three days, of the kind which makes it impossible

---
[27] * As a result of the suggestion.

for either food or drink to pass. This state of affairs gave rise to growing anxiety and fear of death by inanition.

In her infancy the patient had enjoyed good health. Her periods began around the age of 16 and were always regular. At the age of 19 she slipped while skating and fell on her back, hitting her head on the ice. She got up quickly, there was no loss of consciousness, nothing other than contusions along her dorsal spine.

Some time after that she began to experience difficulties in walking which gradually became much worse so that for the last two years she has found herself condemned to a sitting or lying position.

Her arms were also affected and for several months she has been unable to use a needle. No history of hereditary nervous problems.

*Present state.* A well built, well nourished, tall woman, occupying a chaise longue in a half-sitting position.

Her head, trunk and upper limbs are agitated by irregular movements; there is bilateral nystagmus[28]. Under the influence of an effort to respond to a question I pose, the patient's mouth closes spasmodically, her whole body becomes violently agitated, and she only manages to get out a few incomprehensible guttural sounds with great difficulty. After a few minutes rest the agitation in her arms having diminished, she lifts them, one after the other, at my request. However the trembling very quickly resumes and spreads to her trunk and head.

---

28 • Involuntary movement of the eye.

Her legs are rigidly extended, slightly flexed at the knees, her muscles are tense; after some effort I succeed in bending her leg back from her femur, in doing so I observe a tetanic trembling in her crural triceps muscle.

With great difficulty and helped by two people who support her under the arms, the patient manages to get up and take two or three faltering steps. Only the tips of her feet touch the ground. Her feet are turned inwards. All modes of cutaneous sensitivity are preserved.

Her patellar reflexes are exaggerated, sudden dorsal flexion of the foot joints causes clonic contractions of the Achilles tendon. There are no urinary or intestinal abnormalities.

The main symptom worrying both the patient and her family is her inability to swallow.

I quickly succeed in calming the patient and plunging her into a deep sleep. I profit from the state of calm by suggesting the disappearance of the stiffness in her jaws, and persuading her that she could drink a mouthful of water there and then. An attempt to get her to drink immediately succeeds. I assure the patient that she will no longer feel the least difficulty in swallowing.

After about a quarter of an hour I bring her round. She is very calm, feels relieved and remembers clearly and joyously that she has drunk water. She asks for some more and drinks with satisfaction. Her speech is impeded, slow and drawn out, she pauses between each syllable.

The treatment is continued on a daily basis and is followed by a real improvement. After about eight days the patient is able to use her hands and make use of a spoon and fork when eating and drinking. Her sleep which left much to be desired before the treatment has become excellent.

The following 3 August, the patient told me that she had succeeded in threading a needle and had hemmed a napkin. She was able to move her head freely in all directions, without any jerks or tremors, the nystagmus had gone.

Since then the patient's condition has remained stationary, her lower limbs did not benefit from the treatment. I continued to give her a suggestive session twice a week and was thus able to grant the poor girl a state of relative wellbeing.

Now (Dec. 1893), that is to say after more than three years, she has lost none of the advantages obtained through psycho-therapy. For several months she has been complaining of itching in her arms and occasional pains between her shoulders and head. Her general state is satisfactory, the patient is happy. Some inappropriate outbursts of laughter and tears occasionally happen.

That a large place must be reserved for psycho-therapy in the treatment of apoplectic fits is demonstrated once again by observation IV. Electricity and massage achieved nothing, hypnotic suggestion succeeded perfectly in producing a decided improvement in the patient's state.

Fontan and Ségard[29], Bernheim[30], Grossman[31] and others report the same success in similar cases.

## OBS. 4.

LEFT HEMIPLEGIA, FOLLOWING APOPLEXY; IMPROVEMENT.

On the 30 March 1888 a 62-year-old man who had been stricken by apoplexy five years earlier asked to come under my care.

*Present state.* A man of medium height; pale face, dull eyes, labial commissure drooping a little to the left, tongue protruding and trembling, speech impeded; he cries easily. No intellectual impairment. The patient complains of heaviness in his left arm, stiffness in moving his humero-scapular joint and that of his hand, his fingers are held in flexion. The patient can open his hand although it costs him some effort, he closes his fist easily. A tremor occurs on closing his hand.

The left leg is very weak, the patient cannot put any weight on it. He manages to raise it using the support of both arms. His knee is abducted and inwardly rotated so that his foot rests on its outer edge. The patellar reflex is exaggerated.

Occasional urinary incontinence. Defecation retarded. Appetite less than desired. Sleep troubled with nightmares. Some paraesthesia and hyperaesthesia of the left side of the body.

---

[29] Eléments de médecine suggestive.

[30] De la suggestion et de ses applications à la thérapeutique

[31] Dioe Erfolge der Suggestionstherapie bei nicht hysterischen Lähmungen und Paralysen.

Since his apoplectic episode the patient has been unable to walk, he is pushed in a small wheelchair, he despairs of a cure. Electricity and massage have been applied in vain.

After having told the patient's son, in his absence, that the prognosis was very dubious, I undertook treatment at their repeated insistence.

The patient turned out to be very suggestible and easily fell into a deep sleep.

After two weeks treatment, he could walk for a quarter of an hour on flat ground without any help, even without the use of a stick. His sleep had improved and was less troubled by terrifying dreams, his appetite was much better as was his general state of health. No improvement in his arms. The paraesthesia and hyperaesthesia disappeared for only a few hours after suggestion.

This improvement was undeniable.

Suggestions were repeated at infrequent intervals until spring 1891, when a new apoplectic attack was the cause of death.

## A. GROUPE II
# Grand Neuroses
EPILEPSY, HYSTERIA, NEURASTHENIA.

True epilepsy has earned us very little real success. Moreover our results scarcely permit us to advise replacement of treatment with bromides by hypnotic suggestion. In our early trials we used suggestive treatments alone, but we soon had to augment them with bromides.

That is not to say that in some cases suggestion hadn't an excellent effect: with sufficiently suggestible patients we did succeed in reducing the prodromal period a little, in favourably modifying the post-epileptic period, and diminishing the number of fits. However the best results never surpassed those seen during the course of continuing treatment with bromides.

In other neuroses we would only have recourse to this medicine in rare cases, however in the case of pure epilepsy, its continued use seems perfectly justifiable. Should we attribute our setbacks to the fact that in none of our cases were we able to induce a deep sleep? We are tempted to believe it when we compare our results to the brilliant successes obtained by Dr Wettwerstrand of Stockholm. That doctor reports cures of true epilepsy brought about by prolonged sleep.[32]

A definition and meaningful classification of hysterical states and neurasthenia appears to us illusory.

All general definitions of hysteria e.g. that of Benedikt[33]: "an exaggerated disposition of the nervous system to disturbance, either hereditary or acquired", can apply equally well to several recognised syndromes of the neurasthenic order.

It seems to us that we have to accept two or three fundamental pathological states, thus: the aforementioned unstable state of the nervous system; the reduction in power of psychological resistance; and the sense of inferiority usually recognised as a stigma of degeneration. These defective states can combine or present in isolation, or they can transform, according to the individual and the circumstances, into a vast range of other syndromes. And so properly speaking, one has to deal with two or three types of illness, not strictly defined, and at the same time an infinite number of syndromes, a number almost as large as the number of sick individuals.

---

[32] Conf. Zeitschrift für Hypnotismus und Suggestion 1892. S. 17.

[33] Prof. Dr. Moriz Benedikt. Hypnotismus und Suggestion 1894. Eine klinisch-psychologische Studie. S. 71.

Different forms of obsessive ideas, for example, also occur just as often in combination with hysterical and neurasthenic symptoms as they do in an isolated state. It is clear that they arise from a disturbed equilibrium and troubled power of resistance, while the nature of the trouble varies according to circumstances and the particular disposition of individuals. There is scarcely any idea that cannot become obsessive from the moment when normal psychological equilibrium is upset. And if one considers doubting disease and the fear of open spaces as discrete entities, one could go on adding to the number of these conditions indefinitely.

Besides the folie de doute, touching delirium, agoraphobia and claustrophobia, we have had to treat the scrupulous, the superstitious, the fear of storms, of solitude, of travelling, of various illnesses, a heightened sense of guilt, the fear or horror of scars, that of being considered a bad person or being thought to be addicted to sexual perversions, the fear of blushing, of suicide, of homicide, of poisoning one's neighbour, of contaminating or damaging objects and numerous other strange forms of obsession.

Sometimes they present as mild nervous trouble, little different from normal anxiety or non-pathological confusion, sometimes combined with severe psychological disturbance (depression, retardation) or with motor or sensory somatic symptoms.

A characteristic sign can be observed in all these cases, notably a particular idea, impulse, mental state or sensation — which also occurs in perfectly normal people — finds itself insufficiently corrected and counterbalanced and therefore disturbs the patient's mental equilibrium. Most often judgement remains healthy and the patient is perfectly aware of his morbid abnormal state.

Thus from the psychotherapeutic point of view there will need to be — as a general rule with all patients in this category — a consolidation of mental equilibrium and an increase in the power of resistance. It is clear that above all, psychological means are necessary to achieve this end.

Several years ago[34] we maintained that the first concern of the doctor practicing psychotherapy should be to try to increase the psychological stability of his patient. We had no argument with the view that a certain link exists between hysteria and hypnosis or suggestibility, and we thought it could be detected in the psychological dissociation or instability which is innate in the hysteric and artificially induced in the hypnotised.

---

[34] London International Congress of Experimental Psychology, 2nd August 1892. The principles of psycho-therapy by Dr. F. van Eeden.

But at the same time we pointed to the deplorable fact that psycho-therapy — whose theoretical basis was founded by Hack Tuke and who's practical application we learned from Liébault — has been confused and conflated — with hypnotism. In fact the two should be distinguished as clearly as possible.

We are absolutely convinced that the word hypnotism, in Charcot's sense, has nothing to do with psycho-therapy, and only produces confusion.

The only clear and durable way of conceptualising psycho-therapy seems to us to be the following: that psycho-therapy combats illness through the mobilisation of the patient's psychological organ; suggestion, exercise and strengthening through encouragement are its instruments. This conception would surely be seen as an obvious fact, and the most innocent in the world, were it not for the confusion brought about by the abnormal practices of hypnotism.

That it is possible to induce a state of sleep in many patients by verbal influence, and that experience teaches us the influence exercised over a sleeping subject or one half asleep, or in a passive state, acts more powerfully than in the waking state; constitutes moreover a simple fact, not in any way frightening, and is a useful ingredient in the application of psycho-therapy. It permits us to apply psychological therapy methodically.

For the doctor who practises psycho-therapy, hypnotic experiments simply constitute a warning that he could harm his patients if he doesn't stick strictly to therapeutic aims. That is to say he could increase abnormal suggestibility and thus produce an undesirable lasting state of instability, whereas normal suggestibility is absolutely sufficient for his ends, notably cure.

For these reasons we have for a long time kept to the following rules: to never give a suggestion which doesn't conform to physiological facts and to the organism's power of regeneration; to
prioritise as much as possible the centralisation of the psychological organ and to reestablish and reinforce its equilibrium, and thus to act as much as possible in such a way that the healing influence operates through the intermediary of the conscious will of the patient; finally to make use of normal suggestibility but not to exaggerate it any more than necessary.

It seems to us that psycho-therapy understood thus, pure and simple, can resist without fear, even the assaults of a such a violent adversary as professor Benedikt[35] of Vienna.

---

[35] Op. cit.

This academic denies neither the facts of hypnotism nor the effect of psychological intervention on illnesses, demonstrated by Hack Tuke and confirmed by his own observations, but he is vehemently opposed to the methods of the Nancy school. In adopting this position he takes the prize and then throws it away, following the german adage concerning the baby and the bathwater.

One only has to place hypnotic experimentation out of bounds and to gratefully acknowledge that Liébeault has found a simple practical procedure which allows Hack Tuke's theory to be methodically applied. It is absurd to be opposed to a therapy as innocent as this one: the knowledge of how to put a patient into a passive, calm state, with his eyes closed for a period of time, and meanwhile influence him beneficially with words. The question remains: is it effective? To make a judgement we need to gradually collect a large number of observations.

Possible objections, the newness of the method, its imperfections, the chance of a missed diagnosis or omission of a more useful treatment — are all simply things to be borne in mind, but they don't constitute an objection in principle.

A principal component of psychotherapy is the creation of a balance between rest and exercise. It has been studied by

Séguin[36]. He had the happy idea of making patients rest in a quiet place at the same time every day, and then giving them verbal encouragement while doing so. He achieved his success apparently in ignorance of the fact that Liébeault, long before, had put the same principle into practice. Now the method that Dr Séguin followed is, in effect, very similar to the psycho-therapy we have been practising for seven years. But the main component of it all, that is to say the suggestion of sleep followed by verbal suggestion during the sleeping state, wasn't discovered by our American colleague. Without its help, we would have achieved absolutely nothing in the majority of our cases and in the remaining ones, no doubt, achieved even less.

Many patients in the latter group present periods of over-excitation and overactivity and elevated mood, often accompanied by insomnia; alternating with periods of depression, apathy, fatigue and constipation, where sleep is untroubled. In these cases the indications are clear: one should try to reestablish a state of calm equilibrium through prolonged rest during the agitated phase, one should apply a stimulus during the depressive phase.

---

[36] Vorlesungen über einige Fragen in der Behandlung von Neurosen von E.C. Zeugin M.D. in New York.
Ins Deutsche übertragen von Dr. Wallach. Leipzig 1892.

A rigorous diet and seclusion are two other very powerful psychological factors. Together they constitute the basis of the Mitchell cure[37], which we have often made use of with great success while modifying it according to our own views.

In one severe case of hysteria we made use of prolonged sleep lasting five weeks and although it wasn't completely successful, that is to say we didn't succeed in curing the patient, we have to recognise the beneficial effect of the method which puzzled us; we intend to revisit it should a similar case present itself.

**OBS. 5.**

SEVERE HYSTERIA, IMPROVEMENT THROUGH HYPNOTIC SUGGESTION. CURE OF ALL SYMPTOMS AS A RESULT OF PROLONGED SLEEP. RELAPSE.

Miss Z. came to consult me on the 30 August 1888 accompanied by a lady from the town where she worked as a cleaner. She was 37 years of age and unmarried. Her thin, pale face and vacant eyes, imprinted the mark of long suffering on her. Her voice was feint. Since earliest childhood she had been weak and subject to many illnesses. She came without the least enthusiasm and only to please her mistress who had insisted that she try suggestive therapy.

---

[37] * Cure developed by American neurologist Silas Weir Mitchell, usually lasting six to eight weeks. It involved isolation from friends and family. It also enforced bed rest, and nearly constant feeding on a fatty, milk-based diet.

I noted the following facts from her past: Miss Z. was born on 27 Sept. 1851 in a small provincial village to sickly parents. At the age of three years she lost her father who died of Phthisis.[38] Her mother was a hysteric who had epileptic fits from her 21st to 51st year, she died on 23rd Dec. 1885. Of her three sisters, two are still alive; one of them is very nervous, the other is married and healthy, the one who died was stricken by Pott's disease[39]. Her only brother is a drinker.

Too weak to go to school, she learnt to read and write at home. In her early youth she suffered a lot from stomach pains and headaches. At the age of 16 she caught pneumonia. A dry cough and marked general debility dates from that time. She and her family feared that it would become phthisic.

At the early age of 14 she entered a family as a children's nursemaid. Despite being frequently ill, they were happy with her. In fact she spent one out of five days in bed with severe headaches and vomiting. Her menarche didn't occur till the age of 21 after a special treatment had been followed for some time. The doctor looking after her then, told her she would never have normal periods.

As the family in which she served enlarged every year, the patient's duties were negatively affected; her nervous state and her debility increased due to overwork. At the age of 25 she left the service in order to accept a position as cleaner with her present

---

[38] * Consumption or Tuberculosis.

[39] Tuberculous arthritis of the spine.

mistress. During the first three years of her new post (1867 - 1870), Miss Z felt better and did her job faultlessly; however she often had headaches and vomiting during her periods; sometimes they were triggered by overwork or by high summer temperatures.

In March 1869, following an emotional shock resulting from a lover's infidelity, she began to suffer from insomnia and anorexia, intermittent fever, eczema, pemphigus and menorrhagia[40]. After having been treated for a long time with arsenicals, she had two episodes of haematemesis[41]. In 1874 she developed paresis of her lower limbs and contracture of the left leg.

Following a Mitchell-Playfair rest cure lasting 13 weeks, she put on weight but did not regain her strength, she told me that, "A fortnight after the end of my isolation, I lost my voice for the first time". Two days after the cure she was so weak that it was impossible for her to climb stairs and she lost sensation in her upper and lower limbs.

Since that time she has more or less continued to do her job although she has never been free from nervous symptoms, periods of good health alternate regularly with poor ones.

*Present state 30 August* 1888

The patient has suffered from aphony for the last 13 months, she is tired all the time, scarcely sleeps and if she does sleep, her sleep is troubled by terrifying dreams. Anorexia. She suffers from chronic headaches localised at the top of her head, in the

---

[40] * Blistering skin disease and heavy periods.

[41] * Vomiting blood.

superciliary region and behind her eyes. She has not had periods for six months. She frequently passes blood in her urine. Her urine is dark, fetid and there is strangury. Defecation is often slow, she only moves her bowels every 4 or 5 days. When walking she puts more weight on the right leg than the left. The left leg weighs on her and is always tired. When lying down she holds it in semi-flexion; forced extension causes pain in her hip and lower back. She feels tingling in the whole of her left limb. While telling me her history the patient occasionally produces a dry cough. On waking in the morning she coughs a lot, there is no phlegm or saliva but the coughing sometimes provokes vomiting. Once she has vomited she continues, so to speak, to vomit. Most often she brings up a little mucus, sometimes bile and sometimes during recent years, small quantities of blood. She always has a sensation of fullness in the front of her chest, occasional attacks of shortness of breath and fears that her heart is going to stop or of imminent death. She sometimes thinks she has phthisic, sometimes that she is suffering from cancer of the stomach or again a severe liver disease from which she will very soon die. Occasionally she has a transient loss of consciousness unaccompanied by cramps. A symptom which often occurs but mostly in the summer is a vesicular eczema on her hands, feet, neck and the inner side of her joints, it is accompanied by severe itching. Sometimes she presents with hemianopia; rarely both eyes are affected with anopsia[42].

---

42 • Visual field defects.

Examination of the visual organs, and those of hearing, smell and taste is unremarkable; there is anaesthesia and analgesia of the anterior and posterior parts of the lower left limb, an anaesthetic zone the size of the palm of a hand exists in the inter-scapular region. Cutaneous and tendinous reflexes are normal. There is spasmodic contracture of the left leg while lying down. There are no detectable lesions of the thoracic and abdominal organs. Her urine has a specific gravity of 1.021 and contains no abnormal material.

Miss Z. is easily hypnotisable. In her first session she fell into a deep sleep. Appropriate suggestions restored her voice, relieved her headache and corrected her contracture. From that time onwards she attended the sessions assiduously. Most often when she left, she had ben temporarily delivered of the very diverse symptoms with which she continually presented.

Although good somnambulism was achieved with complete amnesia on waking, she only realised my suggestions very fleetingly. Thus her nocturnal sleep didn't improve and her very suggestive dreams undermined the good that my own suggestions had produced. Her condition always worsened at night. She woke up in the morning exhausted and continued her more than heavy duties. She was overtired and didn't eat enough. So long as her state of debility continued her nervous symptoms were finding a propitious soil for development.

However thanks to my treatment, carried out on a daily basis from 30 August 1888 to 12 Nov. 1892, the patient was able to continue her employment, she didn't miss a single day and she abstained throughout that period from medicines which she had previously abused. For about two hours every day, I put her into a deep, calm hypnotic sleep, which restored her for a brief period of time. In short, I helped her a lot but was unable to cure her.

For that reason I suggested to the patient that she be treated with prolonged sleep, basing my advice on the excellent results obtained using this method in cases of hysteria by Doctor Wetterstrand of Stockholm.

She graciously agreed and came into my house where I had a bedroom prepared for her on Sunday 13 Nov. 1892.

A nurse, herself a grand hysteric cured by suggestion, shared her bedroom and never left her side.

*Present state* 13 Nov. 1892, 4 o'clock in the afternoon.

The patient hasn't slept all night due to a severe headache. From 7am to 1pm she hasn't stopped vomiting mucus and bile. She is currently suffering pain in her head, heart and stomach, aggravated by movement. She also feels pain in the hypochondrium and left groin. Contracture of the left leg. This morning semi-liquid stools. Dark fetid urine. Aphonia. Sensation of fullness in the front of the chest.

I get her to undress and go to bed, after which I put her to sleep at 4.45pm.

*Monday* 14 *Nov.* Continues to sleep, no more vomiting. Still a bit of a headache at the top of her head. Feels quite well. Yesterday evening she took a cup of tea and a biscuit before going to sleep. She breakfasted at 9am with tea and a biscuit, towards midday she had some coffee and ate a ham sandwich. Went to sleep at the usual time (3pm) at the polyclinic in my house. In order to do that she had to come down stairs from the third floor, cross over a courtyard and climb another flight of stairs to the first floor.

From then on she did this walk every day, spent one or two hours in the polyclinic and then returned to her room where she took her dinner, still asleep with her eyes closed, and helped by the nurse. Today her dinner comprises soup, a chicken wing and a compote. In the evening she eats an egg.

*Tuesday* 15 *Nov.* Excellent night. Occasionally a few stomach and tooth aches. Urine clear, no deposits. No bowel movement. During the course of the day she takes:

at 8.30am  A cup of tea and bread and jam.

    10am.  An egg.

    midday.  Bread and spread, cold meat, a cup of coffee.

    1.30pm.  A bowl of milk.

    3.00pm.  Some soup.

    6. 00pm.  Some soup, some meat, a vegetable.

    10.00pm.  An egg.

At 5.30pm. finding herself alone for a moment, she wakes up, dreaming of a fire. I put her back to sleep again after about ten minutes.

*Wednesday* 16 *Nov.* During the night she complains of heartburn, she feels like vomiting.

The nurse, breaking with suggestive practice succeeds in calming her. When I see her in the morning the patient blames her headaches on the bad dreams she had. An appropriate suggestion relieves her of the pain and also her aphonia. From then on she became accustomed to speak in a louder voice.

Today's menu is a little fuller than yesterday. The patient is no longer eating against her will.

*Thursday* 17 *Nov.* The night was good. Her voice is clear. The patient is in a good mood, very happy, enjoying her tranquility. She complains of a sticky feelings in her eyes and wonders if this symptom isn't perhaps due to prolonged sleep. An ad hoc suggestion relieves her of the sensation.

*Friday* 18 *Nov.* Her appetite is beginning to grow. Her left limb is completely better, no more contracture, no numbness, no pain, she is supporting herself just as well on the left leg as on the right. Stools normal. From this day onward the patient ate very well, she digested perfectly the average ration for a healthy person of her age. Her strength returned, and her general state of health was excellent. She is satisfied now and is persuaded that her illness is a mental (functional) one, and that she isn't threatened by phisthis, cancer or liver disease.

During the nights of 26 and 27 Nov., she woke up spontaneously with a headache following a dream. The nurse who was asleep didn't become aware of it till 6.30 in the morning. The patient thinks she woke up at 4.30am. The nurse relieved her of her headache straight away and sent her back to sleep.

On 23 Nov. her period began just at the right time, without the least difficulty and finished on 1 Dec. The patient even ate and digested food which she had previously disliked or found indigestible.

On the 2nd Dec. I allowed her to get out of bed at 10am. From then on she went to bed at 10pm and got up in the mornings at 10am. The nurse chats with her and reads the gazette to her. From time to time she has visitors. Everything happens without interrupting her sleeping state. Miss Z. fully enjoys her tranquility and comparing this cure with the Mitchell Playfair one she experienced in the past, she swears that prolonged sleep calms and fortifies in a different way to the isolating cure.

At the end of the 5th week, on Monday 19 Dec., wishing to get the patient used to eating in a state of wakefulness, since she had eaten in a somnambulistic state for the past few weeks, I woke her up just before lunch.

I was deliberately present at this first meal in order to make myself aware of any difficulties that might arise in eating a relatively larger ration, which she was only used to doing in a somnambulistic state. In fact she did raise a few objections which I easily overcame. From that day she continued to eat well. She spent her day doing handwork, reading, chatting and finally taking a walk for 1 or 2 hours. She woke up spontaneously in the mornings at 9am and went to sleep at 10pm in the evening of her own accord, thus acting on a suggestion I had given.

On Sunday 25 Dec. after dinner, the six week cure being finished, she left me in the best of health.

She was absolutely flourishing, with a small embonpoint and rosy cheeks. She couldn't remember a time in her life when she had felt so well.

On saying good bye to her I made her promise to follow the same regime (regarding diet) that she had followed for the previous few weeks and not to relapse into her old ways, that is to say to work beyond the limits of her strength.

For the first week after her cure everything continued to go well. On Wednesday 28 Dec. her period began, was normal and finished on 1 January 1893.

On the following 7 January, Miss Z. developed a fever. A catarrhal angina manifested itself and she lost her appetite, she stopped eating and sleeping well as she had done up till then. Although she came back every day to spend one or two hours in my polyclinic and I did my best to reestablish her equilibrium, my efforts proved to be in vain. Since then her various well known troubles have successively reappeared. The patient continues to do her job, but her state is, alas, the same as before the cure.

*Epicrisis.*

The complete disappearance of all her symptoms both objective and subjective during the prolonged sleep seems to me to evidence hysteria alone as a cause. I dare to say that very probably the patient wouldn't have relapsed if it had been possible for me to continue providing the favourable conditions which she enjoyed for several weeks while in my house. The work demanded of the patient was beyond her physical capacity. Fatigue gave rise to anorexia and consequently a loss of strength and insomnia, and thus the vicious circle formed again, which suggestion alone was unable to break.

The complete cure of chronic headaches in a hysteric who is the object of observation 6, was only achieved thanks to great perseverance. One mustn't despair too early and one must know how to stick with the task in hand. The obduracy of the cure must be opposed to that of the illness.

## OBS. 6.

VIRILE HYSTERIA. CHRONIC HEADACHES. CURE.

A business employee, married man and father of four children, aged 32 years, came to see me on the 17 May 1889 complaining of chronic headaches. He had lost his father at a very young age; his mother was still alive and presented stigmata of hysteria. From his early youth the patient was been subject to headaches alternating with pains in his limbs, said to be rheumatic. Often when the pain is at its maximum he is driven to vomit.

Occasionally the patient has episodes of loss of consciousness accompanied by spasmodic muscular movements of the face and limbs. His digestion is troubled, appetite capricious, bowels retarded.

The patient is often disturbed by globus and pseudo-tympanites[43] of the abdomen.

Two years ago he had a severe lung disease accompanied by intense pain on the right side of his thorax. Since then, although a very thorough examination failed to reveal the least abnormality in his thoracic organs, the patient has occasionally felt the same pains, especially after a cold spell.

Some time ago, he presented with aphonia, a symptom which yielded to electricity.

He has undergone all sorts of treatment for his headaches; although sometimes temporarily relieved, none has been able to cure them.

Most recently he has been prescribed antipyrine which did alleviate them at first at first; however for several weeks this medicine taken at a dose of up to 4 grams had been ineffective. He is frequently unable to go about his business; he also lives in constant fear that one day or another he will lose his job.

He has the occasional good nights, but most often he sleeps badly and has nightmares.

If the headache is severe, he has great difficulty in getting off to sleep, if he does succeed, the sleep relieves his pain.

---

[43] *Lump in the throat and distended abdomen for no apparent cause.

At the end of a bout of headaches, the pain often moves into his arms and legs. These pains are exacerbated by movement. After the pains have subsided his limbs feel blunt and heavy and there is anaesthesia of the skin surface.

There are no objective signs in the various organs.

From the 17 May to 1 June 1889 I gave the patient a session every day. The pains completely yielded to an appropriate suggestion made during a state of light sleep, but they were not slow in coming back to burden him. Also, on the 1June, the patient despairing of the efficacy of hypnotism decided to abandon the therapy. However I succeeded in persuading him to continue the treatment and to good advantage! His sleep became deeper, my suggestions took longer to be neutralised, his pains took much longer to reappear, his nocturnal sleep normalised and his digestion improved. The suggested sleep, light in the beginning, ended up developing into deep somnambulism, and the patient responded in every detail to more or less complicated post-hypnotic suggestions. I continued the treatment for more than a year, giving suggestions every day.

It was only at the end of that time that the patient became completely free of headaches and other morbid symptoms for 3 to 5 days in a row.

Since then I have given sessions at increasingly longer intervals. Today 15 Dec. 1893, a year and a half has gone by since his last session and the cure hasn't been belied. From the 1 June 1889 there hasn't been a single absence from his office.

Observation 7 shows that a diagnostic error can be corrected through psycho-therapy. A patient had been treated for two years according to all the rules of the art for a stomach ulcer. A little afterwards she developed sciatica, resistant to various treatments, which was cured in the end by hypnotic suggestion. This same patient later contracted and was cured of a motley range of nervous symptoms, including symptoms characteristic of round ulcer of the stomach. The latter disappeared as if by magic after several sessions of suggestion, without recourse to a special diet.

## OBS. 7.

SYMPTOMS OF ROUND ULCER OF THE STOMACH FOLLOWED BY SCIATICA. CURE BY HYPNOTIC SUGGESTION. DIVERSE HYSTERICAL SYMPTOMS CURED BY THE SAME TREATMENT AS AND WHEN THEY PRESENTED OVER THE COURSE OF FIVE CONSECUTIVE YEARS.

On the 23rd June 1888 I undertook the treatment of a young 24-year-old woman who had accompanied one of her friends for several days while she was finishing her treatment for a nervous condition.

At first sight one would never have suspected this person, with her air of good health and rosy cheeks, of having suffered from heartburn, haematemesis and chronic sciatica for two years.

She belonged to a group of twelve children of healthy, though nervous parents. One of her brothers was poorly and a drunkard, one of her sisters was a hysterico-epileptic.

She had been vomiting blood for two years. The episodes were repetitive and both preceded and followed by heartburn and pains in the back. She had followed a particular treatment for a long time and although the symptoms of a perforating stomach ulcer had long since disappeared, she continued to follow the *ad hoc* diet originally prescribed.

After the ulcer symptoms had disappeared, those of a right-sided sciatica began. The pain ran from her ischial tuberosity along the posterior and lateral border of her thigh as far as the popliteal fossa and radiated the length of her leg as far as the dorsum of her foot. Locomotion was difficult; the pains varied in intensity; during pain-free periods a sensation of heaviness replaced the pains, exacerbations occurred mainly during the night. The neuralgia had been treated by revulsives[44], electricity and morphine injections.

*Present state* 23rd June 1888

The wellbeing presented by the patient is in flagrant contradiction to her dietary habits. In fact she feeds herself very badly and hasn't the least appetite. No digestive troubles, no heartburn. Sleep leaves much to be desired, neuralgic pains present mainly during the night. During pain-free intervals, dull pains are felt in the right thigh and leg. There are two tender points, notably under the ischial tuberosity and in the popliteal fossa. She has difficulty in

---

[44] • Counterirritants.

walking, which gives rise to pain and tiredness. When walking her foot is internally rotated. No atrophies. Her reflexes are normal. No apparent stigmata of hysteria. The sciatica dates from 12 months ago.

I am able to put the patient into a state of somnolence in a few moments and to relieve her of her pains; even pressure in the tender areas elicits no pain. I encourage her to continue sleeping, and to get up and take some steps. She takes a dozen paces without the least suffering in the world, positions her foot in a perfectly normal way and feels altogether well. I wake her and she leaves satisfied. The pains reappear a half-hour afterwards.

The treatment was continued every day, her sleep failed to deepen, the pains relieved by suggestion recurred sooner or later on the same day.

It was only at the end of January 1889 that the intervals between the pains lengthened (1 or 2 per 24 hours). Since then the sessions have been given at greater intervals. In April the patient was going from strength to strength, she undertook long walks without becoming exhausted. The hypnosis became deeper, and from the 10th July acquired the character of somnambulism with amnesia.

The neuralgic pains were then occurring at intervals of 4 to 6 days, they ceased completely from that time onwards and haven't reappeared to this day (Dec. 1893).

This interesting patient presented again during the course of the years 1889 - 1893 on several occasions complaining of various functional troubles: twice for mutism, frequently for late periods and for headaches, once for haematemesis accompanied by pains characteristic of round stomach ulcer, once for a spastic contracture of the left hand, once for spasm of the eyelid, often for asthenopia[45], twice for constipation and finally once for insomnia.

I always succeeded in reinstating normal functioning within a small number of sessions.

The application of suggestion in cases of repetitive or uncontrollable vomiting has earned us notable success.

## OBS. 8.

UNCONTROLLABLE VOMITING IN A HYSTERIC. CURE.

Young fifteen-year-old girl, slender and anaemic, of non-nervous parents, is the only one of nine brothers and sisters who has nervous troubles. Very small, she presented the phenomenon of merycism[46]; she suffers very often from pseudo-tympanites and digestive troubles. Sometimes she has attacks of heartburn and headaches. She moves her bowels twice a day. Nights are fine. She is normally of a cheerful disposition.

On the 8 August 1891, after having eaten her dinner with a hearty appetite and without the least warning of any indisposition, she vomited the whole lot. The vomiting continued the following day at every meal, the doctor was called who instituted a treatment

---

[45] * Eyestrain.

[46] * Regurgitation of meals followed by consumption.

(crushed ice, bismuth sub-nitrate), leading to a cure. Relapse on the 4th day. A consultation between the family doctor and a specialist got nowhere. Since her condition was worsening the doctor proposed a referral to me.

Finally on the 17th day he accompanied the patient to my consultation.

As the poor girl couldn't keep anything down, even water, her parents were in despair. The patient, on the other hand, wasn't worried at all and scarcely doubted that she would be cured.

Examination by the two colleagues who preceded me in the treatment of this little girl had found an absence of organic lesions and led them to diagnose gastric neurosis, a diagnosis amply confirmed by the success of suggestion in this case.

In the presence of my colleague, I carried out a first session which resulted in the patient being able to keep down some water, drunk in small gulps.

A 2nd and 3rd session enabled her to keep down some whites of egg mixed with water. On the evening of the 4th day of treatment, her mother having been taught by me, profited from the somnolent state of the child, half-awoke her from her first sleep and got her to eat a boiled egg, after which the patient went back to sleep and digested her surprise supper. From the 7th day of treatment the vomiting ceased completely and meals were regularly taken.

More widely spaced sessions were continued until the following 12 Sept. in order to consolidate the cure.

During this time the patient had three nose-bleeds. A stay of six weeks in the country on my advice, put the colour back into the cheeks of the little girl and led to a complete cure.

## OBS. 9.

UNCONTROLLABLE VOMITING IN A HYSTERIC, RESISTANT TO THE USUAL MEDICATION, CURED BY ONE SESSION OF SUGGESTION.

A woman of 40 years. Her father was irascible; her mother suffered a lot with headaches. As a child she was timid, dared not sleep alone. Started having spasmodic nervous fits after puberty without loss of consciousness, alternating with bouts of headaches. She married at the age of 36 years and has two children. No menstrual problems. For two years she has been frequently troubled by abdominal tympanites after her evening meal.

Four weeks ago she started feeling like vomiting when she woke up in the mornings; during the course of the day the nausea disappeared, only to reappear the following day. Her condition worsened and she began to vomit a lot. Soon, every meal was followed by vomiting and the nauseous sensation became permanent. Her doctor suspected an early pregnancy. However her period arrived on time. The treatment instituted did no good and in despair of the cause the patient decided to seek my opinion.

*Present state* 13 February 1890.

The patient, thin, pale, drawn, seems older than her years; she talks volubly and recounts her history in a rambling way; she is anxious. Her breath is fetid. She complains mainly of repetitive vomiting and a continual sensation of heaviness in the region of her stomach; she can't keep down any food or drink, except a little clear water drunk very cautiously. She also suffers from left hemicrania and feels as if there are worms in her abdomen. Bowels move twice a day, liquid. Bad sleep interrupted by tiring dreams. Tongue not coated. Pressure on the sub-xiphoid region doesn't cause pain. Abdominal examination unremarkable.

After having reassured the patient I invited her to sit down in an armchair in front of me. Almost before she had sat down and even before I had made the slightest movement which might have indicated my intention to put her to sleep, her eyes closed. Her respiration became calm and regular. Her skin, completely insensitive to pin prick in different areas, indicated to me that she was in a deep . And so I made some passes along the left side of her head assuring her that the pain was disappearing, then I brought my hand to the top of her stomach and removed the sensation of heaviness. A few minutes later, I woke the patient up. On opening her eyes she emitted a deep sigh and when I asked her how she was feeling, she assured me she was perfectly calm, that couldn't feel any pains and no longer felt any heaviness.

14 *February*. The patient is no longer vomiting, she has been able to eat three small meals and had a good night's sleep. She dreamt that I was hypnotising her. Occasionally the sensation of worms crawling in her intestines still presents itself. I put her to sleep again, repeat the suggestions I gave yesterday, and assure her that

she will not have the uncomfortable sensations described. A 3rd session on the 15 and a final one on the 17 February permit me to consolidate the cure, which is undeniable.

## OBS. 10.

VOMITING OF FOOD IN A HYSTERIC; CURE.

A destitute woman, aged 35 years, widow for two years of a drunken husband, is the mother of five children of whom four succumbed at an early age. The last child left to her is weak and sickly. The patient has always been nervous, she is subject to hysterical fits. At the approach of a fit she feels a strangling sensation in her throat, then she loses consciousness and experiences the need to continually shout and scream. These fits last about 10 to 15 minutes. However they do not worry her and they are not the reason she came to consult me.

A month ago, a scream from her child who felt ill, woke her with a start in the middle of the night. A neighbour called the doctor who judged the case to be very severe and gave little hope to the poor mother. The child is still alive but continues to suffer. From that time onwards the mother has had bad nights, she scarcely dares to sleep for fear that she won't hear her child when he needs her. Rare moments of sleep are troubled with dreams. From the day after that unfortunate night, she started vomiting her meals. To begin with she vomited after every meal, however after a few days she only vomited her dinner.

Her bowel movements are retarded. There are pains in her breasts and under her left shoulder blade as a result of the vomiting. Her breasts are atrophied, not painful to palpation. Her thoracic organs are not affected. Thin weak limbs.

12 Dec. 1893. First suggestive session. Somnolence. Disappearance of pains.

14 Dec. Didn't vomit her dinner. No pains. Light sleep. Suggestive catalepsy.

15 Dec. Yesterday vomiturition[47] after her dinner; however no actual vomiting. She is sleeping better at night. Hypnotic sleep profound.

18 Dec. Everything is back in order. I recommend coming back to see me if the vomiting recurs.

Stopped attending.

Psycho-therapy is often accused of not achieving real cures. Success will only be transient, relapses are the rule. The following observation serves to rebut these accusations. The usual treatments failed to cure a paraplegic, psychotherapy succeeded. A perfect cure was maintained for four consecutive years. During the course of a bout of influenza the paralysis reappeared but was quickly cured again by suggestion.

---

[47] * Repeated ineffectual attempts at vomiting.

## OBS. 11.

HYSTERICAL PARAPLEGIA DATING BACK 12 YEARS, CURED BY SUGGESTION. RELAPSE AFTER 4 YEARS. NEW CURE.

Miss M. was under my care from 6 Nov. 1887 to 10 April 1888. I had the satisfaction of curing her by psycho-therapy of a functional paralysis of the lower limbs which had been present for ten years.

The observation of this case was communicated in our first report, (p. 68 - 70).

In early April 1892, Miss M. contracted influenza and had to stay in bed for several days. It was the first time in four years that she hadn't got up in the morning to take her habitual walk and do the housework. The enforced bedrest, or maybe the feelings of weakness and general debilitation caused by the illness, or perhaps all of these things, probably reawakened in her the idea of useless legs. At least when she tried to get up after several hours of rest in bed, she noticed that her lower limbs refused to work. Although upset by this state of affairs, she wasn't too frightened, convinced that by my treatment she would quickly recover the use of her legs.

She wrote to me from her home (in the provinces) that she was once again paralysed, that the fever hadn't yet subsided and that her doctor had advised her to ask for my care as soon as she was able to travel to Amsterdam. She came on the following 3 May.

*Present state.* The patient has lost her embonpoint, she is pale, feels very weak and is off all food. She has scarcely eaten these last few weeks. She is suffering a lot from violent headaches and complains of pains in her limbs. There is pronounced paraplegia. The patient is in a stuporous state, she has difficulty expressing herself, her speech is impeded, the mucosa at the back of her throat is anaesthetic. The fever has gone. I am aware that she is saturated with potassium bromide.

Having withdrawn all medication I use the first suggestive sessions to improve the psychological state of the patient and relieve her of pain and anorexia. As soon as these problems disappeared I applied myself to restoring movement in the paralysed limbs and instituting methodical exercise in the affected limbs. After four weeks treatment the patient took to her feet, walking wonderfully and finding herself free of all difficulties.

According to her latest news, dated July 1894, Miss M. continues in good health and couldn't be better. She takes a walk for at least two hours every day without the slightest fatigue.

## OBS. 12.

FUNCTIONAL PARAPLEGIA? (ABASIA, ASTASIA)[48] RESISTANT TO VARIOUS TREATMENTS AND ABANDONED AS INCURABLE; NOTABLE PERMANENT IMPROVEMENT BY PSYCHO-THERAPY.

Mrs N.N. is 40 years old, she is married and has a healthy son aged 18 years. As far as I know there is no family history of nervous complaints. She enjoyed excellent health before the year 1886, when she had the misfortune to slip on some stairs. It would be difficult to answer the question: whether the fall was the cause

---

[48] *Inability to stand upright. Lack of co-ordination in walking.

of or a result of the first morbid symptoms which presented themselves around that time.

She lost consciousness after the fall, but regained it a few minutes later and was able to get back on her feet without any assistance. However that accident was followed by a stuporous state. She remembers nothing about it. According to her parents, she was disturbed, had confused ideas, mixed up her sentences and spoke a true galimatias; it was impossible for her to move her limbs, she was incontinent of urine and faeces and had, to say the least, "ataxic troubles". In 1888, she underwent treatment in a nursing home. Her condition at that time was substantially the same. The application of Faradic pincers for ten minutes every day over a zone limited to her arms, restored voluntary movement in her upper limbs so that she was able to do knitting. The same procedure applied to her legs brought no real results. So hypnotic suggestion was tried; however being unable to induce sleep, the treatment was abandoned after eighteen sessions.

Later, electrical treatment was reinstitute under the auspices of a renowned specialist. He took on the treatment with little hope of success, presuming the existence of anatomical brain pathology.

On the 12 Nov. 1889 the patient was entrusted to my care. She is an obese woman, well nourished with rosy cheeks. The expression on her face is vacuous. She replies correctly to simple questions, however she speaks slowly as if in a stupor with a marked tendency to laughter and tears. Her mind is childlike; she is emotionally unstable like an apoplectic. Doubtful paresis of the left facial nerve. She can move her upper limbs and feed herself at mealtimes, however her movements are slow and clumsy. Standing up straight and walking are impossible; she cannot sit down without supporting herself; she cannot turn while lying in her bed. When she tries to get up, assisted by other people, she lets out an imbecilic laugh. The effort is counterproductive. She doesn't make an effort to contribute to any movement she is asked to carry out. However not a single muscle is paralysed. Lying on her back she is capable of reproducing all simple movements shown to her, but it is necessary to insist on this with conviction.

There is diurnal and nocturnal incontinence of faeces and urine.

Sensation is intact. It appears that in the past she has presented anaesthetic zones in the front of her knees. No decubitus.[49] Tendon reflexes are normal. No atrophy nor any diminution of response to faradic electrical stimulation of muscles and nerves.

This paresis is very characteristic. The limbs are inert. If one lifts a hand and one then lets go, the hand remains in the new position and only falls down very slowly. It isn't cataleptic because the rigidity isn't there, it is rather an inertia. The patient forgets the limb, she doesn't understand what one wants of her, she lacks initiative. The voluntary movements that one asks her to carry out are executed slowly. Asking her to lift both arms, she makes the movement, however the right arm more often than not rises before the left. The left leg is also lazier than the right leg. If one asks her to sit down, she always falls onto her right side.

---

[49] • Bedsores.

All movements are possible, but she she doesn't know how to execute them; the idea of coordinated voluntary movement is absent. Movement succeeds better when one explains carefully one's intention and one demonstrates the movement, so she tries to imitate it.

The action of walking is more successful (as I have been able to assure myself during the course of the treatment) when one measures the distance.

She can execute simple movements with her hands, such as the use of a knife and fork when taking meals and knitting. Automatic movements, even slightly complicated ones like knitting, are more successful than movements she has to think about — even when they require a very small expenditure of attention and reflection, such as looking for a particular page in a book. Some longstanding coordinated movements were retrieved intact during the course of her convalescence, whereas the creation of new ones presented great difficulty and had to be studied in the minutest detail.

She had lost the ability to write, and was very satisfied when she succeeded in writing two small very legible notes on 30 Nov. 1889. She relearnt little by little, very slowly, to get up, hold herself erect, and finally to walk, following daily systematic exercise (on coming out of the hypnotic sleep).

From the fourth day of treatment, the patient was able to hold her urine during the night; she could also get herself up and remain standing by pressing her hands down on the back of a chair. On the 30 Nov. the diurnal incontinence of urine was cured and she succeeded in taking a few steps by dragging herself along and holding on to a wheelchair. The least obstacle and any complication in a movement disturbs her, for example deviating from a straight line or turning around. She stops in her tracks and says that she's tired. However there is no lack of muscular force; it's more a question of brain fatigue. As soon as the automatic quality of a complicated movement comes back to her, she becomes indefatigable. (In functional spastic paresis, fatigue interferes with all movements, even those of non-involved muscles).

On the 4 Dec. a small amount of malleolar oedema was present; walking was more difficult. However internal organs were fine and urine examination was negative. The oedema disappeared the following day.

For a long time the patient had complained of pains in her knees, probably caused by unaccustomed exercise.

It would be tedious to describe at length all the details of her convalescence. The hypnotic state obtained by verbal suggestion was adequate. Her suggestibility wasn't great; I wasn't always successful in ridding her of all the pains. I saw the patient every day for at least a year and a half.

In 1890 the treatment was interrupted for about six months, however the patient's condition remained stationary throughout that time. After resuming treatment she continued to make progress. A special diet prescribed for her obesity, contributed to some extent towards the cure. The year went by, I only saw the patient at long intervals.

In order to relearn how to walk she made use sequentially of a wheelchair, crutches, the arms of two people, then of a single person. After that she risked it armed with two sticks, then one, and finally she walked alone.

At the present time (August 1893) she moves about freely in her house, goes from one room to another without support and is able to to take short walks outside on her husband's arm.

Her movements still have a peculiarly clumsy character. She dares not lift her feet enough and the action of turning around is still carried out too slowly and with excessive care.

Her psychological state leaves nothing more to be desired. She no longer exhibits the emotional instability of the past.

The treatment of epileptic fits in hysterics is incumbent on psycho-therapy. In fact psychological means offer much greater chances of cure or improvement in hystero-epilepsy than all other forms of treatment.

**OBS. 13.**

HYSTERO-EPILEPSY; CURE.

Woman aged 62 requested treatment for epileptic fits which had been present for only three days.

She married at the age of 30; before marriage she was subject to epilepsy but since that time the fits had disappeared completely. For several months her health had left much to be desired. She was anxious, neglected her household duties and slept badly at night. She couldn't get off to sleep or else it was troubled by dreams. Often the sensation of a lump rose up from below her navel to the back of her throat, she felt suffocated and felt as if forced to scream.

She yawns all the time, feels agitated and has fleeting pains varying in position and intensity; sometimes in her legs, sometimes in the lower back, or again between her shoulders. Three days ago she suddenly felt a severe throbbing pain in the left hypochondrium, exactly the same as the pain which preceded bouts of cramp in the past. Almost immediately an epileptic fit occurred. These fits have happened five times since then. She consulted a doctor who prescribed potassium bromide.

11 *February* 1892. Abdominal organs unremarkable. The patient goes to sleep easily following verbal suggestion; she enters a profound . I suggest the disappearance of her epileptic fits and the restoration of her sleep at night. On waking after having slept for for an hour, she couldn't remember me having spoken to her.

I repeated the suggestions every day for a fortnight. The fits subsided and calm was restored, little by little, in the course of those two weeks, from the 26 February, the lady was able to resume her housework and no longer complained of anything.

The sessions were then held at greater and greater intervals and the patient left my care perfectly cured at the end of March.

Since then she presented twice more, during the months of May and June, to rid herself of back pains and feelings of tiredness.

Lately (Oct. 1893) I had more news of her. No relapse.

## OBS. 14.

HYSTERO-EPILEPSY, IMPROVEMENT OBTAINED THROUGH SUGGESTION; RELAPSE THROUGH PREMATURE SUSPENSION OF TREATMENT.

An unmarried female villager, aged 27 years, orphaned at a young age and taken in by her grandmother, developed, in her words, "the falling sickness". She has suffered with epilepsy for a long time. More recently the fits have increased in frequency and occurred at night as well as during the day; sometimes up to 4 or 5 fits in 24 hours. Her village doctor has prescribed clear potions with a salty taste

(? bromides) for several years. However she continues to suffer; more recently the same doctor suggested she come to me.

*2 February.* Tall girl with shifty eyes, looks dumb and stuporous, responds slowly to my questions.

She recounts her history in an incoherent way. She stresses one thing, notably that her grandmother cannot get on without her and that she has to get back very soon. No anaesthetic or hysterogenic zones, no other hysterical stigmata. No scars on her tongue. The patient claims that she has never unconsciously urinated during a fit.

I ask the patient to lie down on a chaise longue that I point out, after which I proceed to occlude her eyelids, telling her she will go to sleep. After a few agitated moments, with jerky panting respiration, absolute calm is established and a light regular snore announces that my suggestion of sleep had been realised. So I suggest that she will be free of attacks during the course of the next 24 hours and that the day after her attack will only be a minor one. I bring her round after half an hour's sleep. She opens her eyes, rubs her eyelids, stretches her limbs out lazily and assures me that she has slept well. Complete amnesia.

3 *February*. No fits. While I am examining the patient and asking her a question, spasmodic contractions of the facial muscles occur, her eyes move convulsively inwards and upwards and she suddenly falls on the floor. I immediately take her hand and in a tone admitting no contradiction I order her to get up, assuring her that her head will no longer turn and that she is going to lie down and have a good sleep just like yesterday. She gets up straight away with some difficulty, gives me a far away look, says nothing, stretches out on the chaise longue, closes her eyes and goes to sleep.

Woke up after half an hour feeling very well. During her sleep I suggested that she would no longer have fits.

The sessions were repeated every day and the fits disappeared. However on the 13 February she tells me she felt bad after reading a letter informing her that her only brother, a consumptive, was in danger of dying. She instantly begs me to grant her leave to visit her brother and I agree to the break.

Coming back two days later, I understand that she has been looking after her brother and that feeling very exhausted by the task she had a bout of cramps. After the session she insists on returning home claiming that her grandmother couldn't get on without her. I didn't succeed in dissuading her from the idea. She went home and gave me her news a week later. She hadn't had any fits for the first five days, her brother's condition had got worse, she was watching over him night and day which tired her beyond measure, in addition she had had two fits on the previous night. It was impossible to get her to come back for more care.

I think it isn't too presumptuous to believe that psycho-therapy would have been the correct treatment for this condition had circumstances permitted the patient to leave her milieu and continue the sessions. As it is, she no doubt continued the bromide regime, which wouldn't have cured her and would have put her into an increasingly stuporous state.

## OBS. 15.

EPILEPTIC FITS IN A HYSTERIC. CURE ACHIEVED IN A SINGLE SESSION OF SUGGESTION.

A young man aged 21 years, thin and malnourished, son of a hysterical mother and a neurasthenic father, consulted me on 6 Oct.

1891, accompanied by his father whom had been under my care for some time.

He is very irritable, has always had a nervous disposition but has never had nervous fits. Six weeks ago, after a fit of temper, he broke into alternating bouts of laughter and crying, which were followed by generalised trembling, clacking of the teeth, then tonic and clonic spasms with loss of consciousness. After about an hour the patient regained consciousness. Since then, these fits have been repeated several times. The father who observed them assured me that they were exactly the same as his mother's fits in every detail.

After having put the father to sleep in the presence of his son, I invited the latter to sit down and on closing his eyes I suggested sleep and the disappearance of his symptoms. I woke him after about twenty minutes. He gave the impression of having been aroused from a deep sleep and couldn't remember that I had spoken to him.

I haven't seen this patient again, but his father whom I continue to see from time to time, assures me that the epileptic fits have not recurred.

**OBS. 16.**

EPILEPTIC FITS IN A HYSTERICAL MAN; CURE.

An unmarried man aged 27 years that I treated for a paresis and pains following severe rheumatic arthritis, and cured with hypnotism (Sept. to Dec. 1887), came to consult me on 4 Nov. 1889.

He belongs to a nervous family. His mother and one of his sisters are hysterics.

The patient is an extremely irritable man. The previous day after a fit of anger he burst into bouts of laughter and crying followed by loss of consciousness and clonic contractions. The seizure lasted for about a quarter of an hour after which he slept for an hour and a half.

The fit of anger was preceded by headaches (a symptom that often troubled him), strong throbbing in his temples and an unaccustomed sensation of sadness. It's the first fit of this kind that the patient has had. He had a bad night with horrible dreams. He felt run down, depressed, incapable of either working or reading.

Five days of treatment sufficed to restore the patient to his normal state.

I saw him again a year later, notably on 6 Oct. 1890. He came to ask me to rid him of a (rheumatic?) pain in his left arm. A single suggestion corrected the problem. I learnt on that occasion that the hysterical fits had not recurred.

## OBS. 17.

HYSTERO-EPILEPSY, TIC DOULOUREUX, CURE.

On the 2nd May 1892 Mr D. asked me to come and care for his wife who had nervous attacks and suffered from tic douloureux.

*Family history.* Mrs D. is the daughter of a hysterical mother, she has two very nervous sisters.

*Personal history.* Before her marriage the patient suffered from headaches, dyspepsia, globus hystericus, pseudo-tympanites and vertigo. These symptoms continued to occur after the marriage. Following an abortion, Mrs D. had a first attack of epilepsy. The fits subsequently occurred when she was emotionally stresssed. Her husband's condition, above all, caused her a lot of anxiety and worry. In fact Mr D. is consumptive and has had an haemoptysis[50] on a number of occasions.

Some months ago the patient had a toothache and several decaying teeth were extracted. However the pain didn't get better and gradually took on the character of neuralgia. Since then terrible spasms of tic douloureux have added to her other woest, rendering her life unbearable.

The family doctor exhausted his ability to help the patient and advised her to consult me as a last resort.

*Present state.* Mrs D. is in bed in the middle of a spasm; the pains are in the left side of her face, they radiate from the mastoid apophysis towards her eye, cheek, mouth and chin. During the day she has had several epileptic fits.

While the husband is explaining his wife's case to me, I sit down next to her and taking her hand in mine I ask her to close her eyes, saying that I am going to put her to sleep and take her pain away. Continuing to exert light pressure on her eyes, I affirm the sleep

---

[50] *Coughed up blood.

and then set to making some passes over the painful areas. Calm is soon established, the patient ceases to moan, her respiration becomes regular, she relaxes and a deep sleep overtakes her. I assure her that she feels very well, that her pain is dissipating, that she is going to have a good night, that the epileptic fits will become few and far between, and that tomorrow in the afternoon at one o'clock she will find herself well enough to come to consult me. After several minutes I leave the patient following a final suggestion, notably that she will wake up spontaneously in half an hour and be pain free.

3 *May* 1892. At 10 o'clock in the morning the husband arrives to beg me to allow his wife to come immediately, because she feels an epileptic fit will happen if she has to wait till one o'clock in the afternoon.

She had a good night but on waking the neuralgic pains had returned. I told Mr D. that I could only receive his wife at the appointed time.

At one o'clock in the afternoon I was informed that Mrs D. was in the waiting room and that she was having a fit. I immediately went to her side and in a forceful tone ordered her to calm down immediately, to get up and accompany me upstairs to the first floor, where she would find a chaise longue that she could use. So saying, I took her hand. She got up straight away, accepted my arm and came with me. Once settled on a sofa I put her to sleep and let her sleep for the next two hours, suggesting in the intervening time the complete disappearance of her tic and her epileptic fits. Before bringing her round I assured her that she would feel so well that on waking she would send the carriage away and go home by foot, a suggestion which she in fact carried out to the letter.

4 *May* The patient comes at the same time to ask for a session. She is radiant, blissfully happy that her pains have not recurred.

I continued Mrs D.s treatment until October with much success. Her general state of health gradually improved, various nervous symptoms responded to appropriate suggestions. On one occasion the tic occurred again and she had a hysterical fit precipitated by her husband spitting blood. The prosopalgia[51] responded definitively to suggestion after I had extracted, under hypnotic sleep, three tooth roots that I found on examining her mouth.

On the following 8 Oct., I was called in haste to the patient's side, who had become very ill. Mr D. had died suddenly during an episode of copious haemoptysis. I found the patient in a worrying stuporous state of apathy. It was only after several hours that I succeeded in drawing her out of her state of despondency and mournful sadness. She allowed her tears flow, let herself get undressed and go to bed at my urging. A sleep of several hours relieved her a little.

Following that catastrophe Mrs D. developed symptoms of melancholia with suicidal ideation which lasted for about a month. Thanks to the influence I had over her, thanks to my repeated suggestions and to the hypnotic sleep, I was able to chase away the black ideas and I had the satisfaction of seeing my interesting

---

[51] Trigeminal neuralgia, tic douloureux.

patient completely cured. Since then I have seen her from time to time at increasing intervals. She continues to be perfectly well. Neither the epileptic fits nor the prosopalgia have recurred. The latest news dates from February 1894.

The patient who is the object of the following observation was subject to hysterical fits in her childhood. For a long time she led a life which although laborious was without worries, her health left nothing to be desired. From the moment that she saw herself deprived of a master on whom she had relied until then, she lost confidence in herself and the latent hysteria came to the fore.

**OBS. 18.**

VIRILE HYSTERIA. OVERWHELMING ANXIETY STATE IN A PATIENT WHILE CARRYING OUT HIS PROFESSIONAL DUTIES, IMPOSSIBILITY OF CONTINUING HIS EMPLOYMENT. CURE IN SEVERAL SESSIONS.

A butcher's boy aged 25 years asked me to rid him, if possible, of a nervous condition which had been bothering him for some time and which he thought was threatening to cost him his job.

He lost his parents at an early age and knows no other family. He is aware that he has always been very nervous and claims to have often had breakdowns. In fact because of these breakdowns he was kept away from school. At the age of 16 years, he entered the service of a master-butcher. From that time, the nervous bouts no longer occurred. He enjoyed learning his profession and never felt the least difficulty nor repugnance during the slaughter of animals or the exercise of his duties. He always served the same master. When this master died, several months ago, he took over the management of the business under the patronage of his widow.

Now, for some time he has lost his normal state of mind, he feels ill at ease when he has to slaughter an animal. Whereas before he cut the throat of an animal with sang-froid at his master's command, this has now become impossible for him. Even the idea of having to use the knife produces a sense of strangulation in his throat. If he wants to strike he feels as if his throat is caught in a vice, his neck begins to hurt, a nervous cough occurs which becomes more and more forceful and calm is only reestablished after relinquishing the work. The coughing fit ends with the production of some mucous. If he persists in continuing work, he is overtaken by vertigo and an indescribable anxiety renders him incapable of making a movement. Apart from a few pains he feels from time to time between his two shoulders and on the front of his chest, the patient enjoys good health.

Local examination demonstrates the absence of objective signs. The patient isn't a drinker and is not debauched. He feels disheartened and begs me to cure him. If he doesn't get better he will be forced to leave his job.

Without further ado I abruptly proceed with the occlusion of his eyelids after having promised that I would cure him, and I confirm that he is asleep. Taken by surprise, the patient begins to shout like a madman and starts trembling and has a hysterical fit.

In a forceful and imperious tone I order him to be silent, to have breath calmly and to continue to sleep easily.

The patient obeys instantaneously, calm prevails and he falls into a deep sleep. He doesn't feel pin pricks that I make in his arm. I lift his arm and defy the patient to lower it; the arm remains elevated in catalepsy. I now formulate the suggestion that he will no longer have any anxiety and that the nervous symptoms which preceded and accompanied that state will no longer occur, that he will recover the cool head he had in the past and that he will once again happily carry out all the jobs necessary in the slaughterhouse. I let him sleep for a quarter of an hour then wake him up. He rubs his eyes looks at me astonished, doesn't know where he is, then he remembers that he had come to consult me, that he had told me his story, but the rest escapes him.

The following day 12 *Sept.* he comes back to see me. I give him a quarter-hour session. This time he goes to sleep without the slightest agitation. I repeat yesterday's suggestions.

13 *Sept.* The patient is very happy. Yesterday he slaughtered a cow and did the whole job without the least agitation. He feels cured and thanks me effusively.

In order to consolidate the cure I gave four more widely spaced sessions to this young man. No relapse.

A cardinal point in psychological treatment is certainly to know how to gain the confidence of the patient, to show him sympathy, to listen patiently to his complaints, to prove that you are interested in his suffering and troubles. Another point is to provide a comfortable milieu away from everything that could interfere with the suggestive process to which one is going to subject him, so that anything that could irritate him or remind him of his troubles is far away.

In observation 19 the patient, despite having followed a psychological treatment conducted by the family doctor, only began to clearly improve after changing to a more propitious environment, a change which our colleague himself had advised.

## OBS. 19.

SEVERE NERVOUS ATTACKS OF A HYSTERICAL TYPE; CURE.

A colleague practicing in the country asked me to care for one of his clients whom he had treated since the beginning of January 1892 for nervous episodes of a hysterical type.

It concerned a young 23-year-old girl, tall, slender but thin and flat chested; her mother died of pulmonary phthisis and her brother has just died of the same condition. Her illness began with fits of clonic spasms principally affecting her four limbs and accompanied by pains in the neck and face. Then her legs became paralysed and the patient found herself condemned to stay in bed. Concomitant symptoms; minimal catarrh of the apices of the lungs, habitual constipation and irregular periods. A treatment by suggestion instituted by the doctor, combined with treatment with bromides produced a satisfactory result. At least, after several weeks the patient was in a state where she could get up and walk a few paces whilst leaning on the arms of a couple of people. She paid her first visit to me on 13 April 1892.

Tired from a four hour steam-boat and rail journey, she descended from the carriage with difficulty and it was only with the support of two people that she could take the few steps necessary to enter my consulting room. Having come in, she let herself fall into, rather than sit, in a large armchair.

It was only with great difficulty that she brought herself to respond to the questions I addressed to her during my examination. The reason was a state of partial trismus[52] which prevented her from opening her mouth properly. Her brother, who accompanied her, assured me that recently the patient had been feeling low, melancholic, and that she burst into tears for no reason and scarcely ate; primarily because she wasn't in the least hungry but also because she could hardly unclench her jaws, so she only lived off a little milk. The poor girl is excessively thin, she hasn't, so to speak, any skin on her bones. She doesn't sleep at night, coughs from time to time but doesn't bring anything up. She complains of pains in her jaws, in her neck, in her back and in the front of her

---

52 * Lockjaw.

thorax, a general lassitude and continual tiredness in her legs; finally she has slow bowel movements and has had amenorrhea for fifteen weeks.

On examination of her chest I noticed a slightly resonant clear sound under both her clavicles, but mostly on the right side, a less resonant sound in the posterior apices, whistling respiration without râles in the anterior and posterior apices, normal elsewhere.

The pain in her neck radiates toward her jaws and towards the front of her chest. Several molars and several other teeth are decayed. There are no sensory problems.

During my examination I succeeded in winning the confidence of the patient who made me understand that family distress had been the point of departure for her illness. I was able to calm her, I found consoling words, I promised her my assistance in dealing with certain difficulties that she believed insurmountable, after which I succeeded perfectly in putting her to sleep. She left me feeling very calmed and promising to come back the following day.

From then on she came to see me every day. All her symptoms successively got better and her strength returned. At the beginning of the 3rd week she had the courage to have all her decayed teeth extracted; from that time on the pains in her neck and jaws plus the trismus disappeared completely. Her menstrual periods returned, the anorexia gave way to a perfectly normal appetite and from the 14th day of my treatment the patient found herself able to take an hour long walk on her own.

On the 8 May I granted her leave for a few days to go and see her family.

On her return, I continued the sessions which from the 15 June were given at increasing intervals, until her complete recovery. The patient left the clinic, cured, on 10 July.

In Sept. 1892 she gave me excellent news of her health and made me aware of her marriage plans. The wedding took place on the 17 Sept. following.

Asked by the patient who is the subject of observation 20, to rid him by suggestion of a persistent and tiring hiccup, I thought that a meaningful and lasting cure demanded a no less meaningful treatment of his general state. Before anything else a change of milieu was mandatory in this case. After a change of diet to which the patient was subjected, his general condition soon improved, the hope of a cure was reborn, and the suggested sleep restored his shaken equilibrium. Most of the time the patient didn't respond to direct suggestions, other than that of sleep; rather the cure was obtained by daily repetition of prolonged sleep for three and a quarter hours, and by more general suggestions of calm and wellbeing.

## OBS. 20.

ANOREXIA, INSOMNIA, PERSISTENT HICCUP IN A HYSTERIC. NOTABLE IMPROVEMENT. RELAPSE AFTER 9 MONTHS. RESUMPTION OF TREATMENT FOLLOWED BY CURE.

An unmarried lady, aged 43 years, residing in a provincial town presented nervous symptoms from her tenderest age. Her very large family includes several hysterical and neurasthenic members. The family doctor treated her for nearly a fortnight for an intractable hiccup. A recommendation on his part to try treatment by suggestion was accepted and I was asked to come and see the patient.

On the 21 Sept. 1890 I found her, lying in her bed, in a state of extreme weight loss, her whole body shook continuously from a painful hiccup which reminded me of a dog barking. She could only speak in a jerky way with continual interruptions. A potion of chloral was within reach. From hour to hour she took a spoonful which gave her a few minutes respite. She had the hiccup night and day. Ordinarily a small eater, she had eaten absolutely nothing for the last few days. Her legs were paralysed. This condition of the lower limbs had been present for several months, and was moreover a symptom with which she was familiar and which had often affected her for a greater or lesser period of time.

On examination I elicited ovarialgia on the left side, a hyperaesthetic zone in the lower back and general hyperaesthesia of the four limbs. No anaesthesia. She often had little hysterical fits without loss of consciousness, preceded by globus. Otherwise nothing abnormal.

I indicate to the patient that her condition, although serious, doesn't present a grave danger, but that special treatment in my clinic is absolutely necessary to cure it. Although desirous of following my advice, the journey (2 to 3 hours by rail) put the poor lady off and she feared she wouldn't be able to tolerate the fatigue. I reassured her, suggested (without putting her to sleep), that she would have a good night and would be able to make the journey on the following day. Upon which I retired.

22 *Sept.* 1890. In fact the patient slept for 3 or 4 hours after my departure, and managed the journey without undue difficulty. On arriving at my clinic she lay down immediately, ceaselessly disturbed by her hiccup.

Placing my hand on her forehead I easily succeeded in putting her to sleep. I made use of the calm thus produced to suggest a good night's sleep and the disappearance of her disgust for food. I let her sleep for an hour. On awakening, she felt better, although the hiccup continued from the moment she awoke. Milk diet. In the evening at 10 o'clock I put her to sleep again and left her sleeping.

23 *Sept.* Apart from two breaks, each of about one hour's duration, the patient slept through the night. The hiccup continued from the moment she woke up. Heartburn, frequent eructations. At the request of the patient, I hypnotised two other patients in her presence, a spectacle which greatly interested her. Immediately afterwards I put her to sleep and suggested the gradual

disappearance of her hiccup. In the evening at 9 o'clock, another session, followed by a prolonged sleep without interruption until 6 o'clock in the morning.

24 *Sept.* The hiccup is much less marked and there are long periods of respite, the patient is less depressed, gains in confidence, she is drinking her milk without aversion. One 3 hour session in the afternoon does her so much good that she isn't disturbed by her hiccup throughout the evening. Her ration of milk is gradually being increased.

1 *Oct.* Over the last few days the patient has made real progress. The hiccup only occurs occasionally for about quarter of an hour. She sleeps 2 to 3 hours during the day and enjoys a good sleep the whole night long. She is gaining in strength. *Diet*: 2 eggs and 2 litres of milk every day.

11 *Oct.* Has been able to leave her room, she feels that her strength is returning, is less weak in her legs. Today she dines at the table for the first time with my family and the other patients. *Diet:* Bread, two eggs, three litres of milk and a whole dinner. No longer melancholic at all, gaining a small embonpoint. The hiccup has disappeared completely for 2 or 3 days at a time. When it does happen, it doesn't last more than 10 minutes. I taught the patient how to get rid of it by auto-suggestion.

22 *Nov.* The cure is more and more established. The patient is already taking walks lasting between one and one and a half hours without getting tired.

She feeds herself very well although lacking in any real appetite. She has put on 7 kilogr. in weight since her arrival. The hiccup still occurs sometimes but infrequently, mainly when she is tired or when she becomes emotional. The patient always succeeds in ridding herself of the symptom by lying on a chaise longue; she goes to sleep in that position so that the hiccup disappears, and after about a quarter of an hour she wakes up feeling refreshed. She is no longer in the clinic but will still be coming to see me from time to time until the end of December. Having returned home on 1 January 1891 she wrote me this letter on the following 18 February:

Dear doctor,

" I deliberately waited for some time before giving you my news, which is excellent. I waited in order be able to assure myself that my cure was really secure and that it wasn't just a temporary improvement. Now I am no longer holding back and I thank you with all my heart for the good care that you provided for me. I will be grateful to you for the rest of my life.

My family finds me so much changed for the better that they cry miracle, etc. etc."

The same patient presented again on the 23 Oct. 1891, at first for hysterical trembling in the right leg, then the left lower limb, together with hyperaesthesia of the skin from below the armpit to the right knee, and for a sensation of general weakness. For several weeks she had been sleeping less well at night and felt herself repossessed by an aversion to food. Also, she was occasionally disturbed by a slight bout of hiccups. It seemed to her that autohypnosis was succeeding less quickly and less well than previously in vanquishing this symptom.

Once asleep, she showed an exaggerated sensitivity even to the very light passes I made in order to try and calm her trembling. She seemed completely refractory to my direct suggestions. From then on I contented myself with prolonging the sleep for 3 to 4 hours, without making any suggestions during that time. I limited myself to assuring her that sleep alone would would cure her. I repeated these sessions at first thrice, then twice a week until 1 May 1892. On that date the patient once again felt perfectly recovered and free of her various symptoms.

Since then I have had news of her from time to time which continues to be excellent.

## OBS. 21.

CONTINUOUS LARYNGEAL CHOREA IN A HYSTERIC, PERSISTING FOR TWO YEARS, CURED BY HYPNOTIC SUGGESTION.

A well-rounded, plump woman about 40 years old, with a stuporous air, came to see me on the 8 February 1893.

She came in coughing paroxysmally, with a raucous cough reminiscent of the sound produced by a seal, and brought a handkerchief alternately to her mouth and neck. A relative who accompanied her asked me to examine her. Speaking tired the patient and her companion gave me the clarifications I requested. For two years previously the patient had been tormented by this continuous cough and all attempts at treatment had failed. There are many nervous people in her family. She herself paid a large tribute to different nervous illnesses. She often had headaches, a lump which rose up from her stomach to her throat, stomach problems and also fits of nervous convulsions. The patient complained of pain in the larynx and felt a sensation there, as if something was out of place. It was impossible for her not to cough. Her respiration was accelerated and breathless; she calmed down during sleep, became normal and the cough ceased, only to continue when she woke up. Examination of her airways revealed no organic lesion.

One of my colleagues, a specialist in laryngeal diseases to whom I referred the patient for assessment, confirmed the normal state of her larynx and asked me to leave the patient with him for a few days so that he could try out some medication that had given him brilliant results in similar cases. I willingly abandoned the patient and she was submitted to the action of antipyrine. However after three weeks he sent her back to me, coughing just as before.

On the 22 February I began treatment by suggestion. Having made her sit down in an armchair, I closed her eyelids and affirmed sleep. After several seconds her noisy respiration became calm, she stopped coughing and fell asleep. I suggested to her that the repetition of my treatment would gradually bring a cure, that she would regain her capacity to resist the irritation caused by the cough, finally that gradually the pain in her neck and the sensation of displacement that she felt would diminish and disappear.

Woken after half an hour, she replied to some questions that I posed without coughing, she felt less pain, felt calm and believed that she would get better. Several moments later, as she was putting on her hat, the cough reappeared.

I continued the sessions on a daily basis and after a fortnight I was able to assure myself that a notable improvement had been produced. In place of a continuous cough, the phenomenon only now occurred at intervals which grew longer and longer. She felt strong enough to control the cough when she wanted to. The pain in her neck was diminished but not yet completely absent. She felt better and happy with the progress she had made.

Towards the end of March, the patient was only coughing occasionally. Sometimes she enjoyed deliberately provoking the vanished symptom to demonstrate her problem when in the waiting room recounting her troubles to other patients. From the moment that I appeared and surprised her during this little performance, she became flustered and full of excuses and suppressed her cough immediately.

As and when the cough disappeared, the patient began to suffer from her headaches and dyspeptic symptoms.

From 1 May to the end of July I saw the patient at greater intervals. She is keeping well and is only bothered by her cough after forceful exercise or strong emotion. She knows how to suppress the phenomenon quickly by saying to herself mentally: "The doctor has forbidden me, I don't want to cough anymore."

Towards the end of August I received a letter of thanks from the patient. She expressed her gratitude and said that she was cured.

However I saw her again on the following 23 Sept., coughing more than ever. She informed me that after having been free of her cough for six consecutive weeks she had been afflicted by the death of her father, and the cough had reappeared since then. A few sessions quickly corrected the phenomenon and the patient continues to be well. (August 1894).

## OBS. 22

TREMBLING AND FITS OF ERUCTATION IN A HYSTERIC. CURE.

A poor 40-year-old woman, married at the age of twenty but abandoned by her husband long ago and maintaining herself with difficulty, came to consult me on the 29 Dec. 1891.

Of her past history she was only able to tell me that at the age of 17 she had been knocked over by a carriage and that the accident had triggered a hysterical crisis. Finally that for more than a year she had been treated for a melancholic condition.She had no further information to give me.

The poor woman brought me up to date with her suffering in tears. She had had sleepless nights for a long time, she got up in the mornings in order to go to work feeling tired, and came back in the evenings even more exhausted. She had no appetite, ate little and badly. She was fearful and subject to bouts of trembling, sometimes lasting for more than an hour. Another symptom that bothered her a lot was a noisy eructation which came in fits which could surprise her at any moment, and which she knew could be easily set off.

On examination I discovered nothing abnormal. Before hypnotising her, I got her to watch the treatment of some other patients. Her turn came, I began to close her eyes and put her to sleep; however she became anxious, her thoughts were elsewhere, and instead of the desired sleep, the noisy eructations emerged.

Raising my voice, I ordered her to stop the racket straight away. Almost instantaneously she obeyed, but at the same moment she began to tremble all over her body. So I softened my voice, reaffirmed that sleep was going to come, that she already felt calmer, that the trembling was beginning to go away, that it would decrease little by little, that she would soon no longer tremble at all, and finally that she was asleep. And in fact, over the course of a few minutes, she was indeed overcome by a peaceful sleep. I made use of it to give the necessary suggestions. I saw the patient again the following day. She had slept from one o'clock at night until seven in the morning, felt much better, was no longer crying and was less tired. No eructation. No trembling.

31 *Dec.* The patient slept all night. The improvement persists.

13 *Jan.* 1892. Today the patient that I had seen again three times over the last few days came to take her leave. No further complaints.

## OBS. 23

DIFFERENT FUNCTIONAL PROBLEMS, PRESENTING OVER THE COURSE OF THREE CONSECUTIVE YEARS IN A HYSTERIC, CURED BY SUGGESTION.

It concerns a 43-year-old unmarried lady of good constitution. She consulted me for the first time on the 8 July 1889, complaining of having become deaf, or at least hard of hearing for several months. Cared for at first by her regular doctor, then by a specialist, these gentlemen had assured her that there was nothing wrong with her auditory organ and that the problem was functional. The patient feeling that they were too dismissive of her case, came to ask my advice.

On examination I noted perfectly normal hearing and the absence of organic lesions of the auditory organ. The patient recognised that in fact, properly speaking she was not deaf. It was just that when someone addressed a word to her, she didn't hear it or heard it badly, because her attention was distracted by noises in her ear and head. Sometimes they are like the noise of waves, other times she hears church organ music, or even bells chiming, or again the dull rhythmical sound of a mallet hammering in posts.

She hears the sounds mostly in her left ear, sometimes it the seems to come from outside her head, from a point situated just above her left ear; however occasionally the right ear is also involved. These sounds disturb her and stop her from sleeping or concentrating on anything.

There is a family history of nervous problems. In her personal history I learn that she presented with aphonia, weakness in the hands and forearms so that she couldn't hold anything, and finally paresis of the lower limbs.

A treatment by suggestion begun on the same day, resulted in the complete disappearance of the main symptom and consequently that of the secondary symptoms, namely agitation and insomnia. The cure was completed at the end of August.

In Sept. 1890, the lady presented again and asked me to rid her of an incessant cough which had been tiring her for several days and appeared refractory to her normal doctor's medicine. Four sessions of suggestion in a deep sleep sufficed to bring about a cure.

In April 1891, I saw my interesting patient again. This time she complained of tiredness and heaviness in her left leg, of a garter like sensation above her knee on the same side (it should be noted that she never wears garters). Cure in three sessions.

On the 24 April 1892, the patient told me that in the last few months her periods had been irregular. She had not had a period for thirteen weeks, but when they were due she was disturbed by vertigo, heartburn and vomiting. That state of affairs lasted three or four days, then disappeared. I put the patient to sleep and confirmed her state; I suggested to her that the nervous symptoms would no longer happen, that it was possible that the menopause was beginning, but that when it did she would no longer be troubled. My suggestion was perfectly realised. Since then the patient has given me good news from time to time.

## OBS. 24

TINNITUS AND DIVERS NOISES IN THE EARS; CURE BY HYPNOTIC SUGGESTION.

Mrs B. L., married and aged 68 years, had been nervous all her life without ever presenting serious problems. Following a head cold accompanied by repeated sneezing, she developed continual tinnitus in both ears but mainly in the left one, a symptom which worried her. The care which her ordinary doctor gave her didn't help. The diagnosis, made by a specialist she consulted, concluded there were no organic lesions and the trouble was nervous and functional.

On the 4 January 1892 the patient came to see me. I understood that she was worried beyond measure by a noise that she could hear night and day. She heard it continually like a doorbell being rung all the time, and intermittently she heard the monotonous sound of bells and some shouts in the road. In addition movement of her head made her hear the rhythmic sound of sleigh-bells. These sounds were located inside her head but varied in position. Waking up from a period of sleep the concert immediately continued. She was obsessed with it. Cheerful and lighthearted before her her cold, the good lady had become somber and irascible, refused to eat, took no interest in anything, preferred to die rather than continue to live that way.

Normally constipated, she purges herself every day.

On examination I find no hysterical stigmata nor any organic problems.

I succeed in calming the patient by citing examples of nervous states like hers which have been cured by suggestion and I manage to hypnotise her without too much difficulty. Once asleep, I suggest that she will have better nights, that the sounds will gradually disappear, that they will seem to come from further away and get softer and softer, that during sleep she will no longer hear anything. My prediction came to pass in short order and in the course of three weeks she felt much better. She slept well at night, regained her good humour and although she still occasionally heard the sounds during the day, she was scarcely worried about them. Just then on 22 January she fell ill with influenza and had to interrupt her treatment.

The sessions were not resumed until the following 29 February. Having disappeared completely for some time, the noises had made their reappearance during her convalescence. However the patient wasn't as worried about them as she had been previously and was sure that my suggestions would right the situation.

The treatment continued until the 14 June. At first I saw the patient every day, then at intervals more or less close according to how she was feeling. The symptom soon disappeared completely and during her stay in the country, where she spent the summer, Mrs B. L. was n't at all troubled.

Treatment was resumed at the beginning of the following September. The noises were triggered by emotional states or any intercurrent indisposition, but they were no longer continuous and she was much less obsessed by them. The patient complained more of bad dreams, vertigo and loss of appetite.

These diverse symptoms were improved or suppressed completely by appropriate suggestions.

The cure was lasting. The latest news dates from July 1894.

## OBS. 25

FITS OF ANGER AND BAD HUMOUR IN A HYSTERIC. CURE BY HYPNOTIC SUGGESTION.

One of my patients, a hysterical lady with mixed attacks whom I had been treating successfully for some time with suggestion in a state of somnambulism, asked me if she could bring her niece whose bad humour was causing a lot of upset in the family. Very irascible, the niece got edgy over nothing and after a fit of anger spent entire days sulking. Perhaps, my patient thought, suggestion could effect some improvement in her bad behaviour and cure her of her outbursts.

On 8 April 1890 I met her niece, a small brunette aged 22 years. She looked well, excellent constitution and seemed to enjoy a good state of health. She confessed that she felt sad and irritable all the time, that she suffered a lot with headaches. Just then she had pains in her lower back, in her kidneys and was affected by a tremor in her right hand.

There were many nervous people in her family, mainly hysterics. She submitted herself willingly to an examination which revealed no organic lesions.

After having put to sleep several patients in the presence of the newcomer, I suddenly turn to her and order her to go to sleep. I look into her eyes with a fixed stare. Almost instantaneously her eyelids begin to twitch, her eyes roll upward, she sleeps. I make her sit down and confirm for myself by pricking her arm that she is analgesic; on raising the limb it stays fixed in that position. Then I proceed to formulate an appropriate suggestion first regarding the disappearance of of her pains, then also of the tremor. The latter symptom disappears immediately after the order is given. She replies negatively to my question as to whether she still feels pain anywhere. And so I risk just asserting that from that moment she will find herself a completely changed character. Her black moods will no longer exist, she will from then on be cheerful and no longer get carried away, she will be sweet and amiable with everybody. I add that the hypnotic sleep is very agreeable to her and that she would like to experience it again. I let her rest for a quarter an hour more, then I wake her up. Complete amnesia.

I review the young lady the following day, she is very well, doesn't have any pain but expresses the desire to be put to sleep again. The aunt confirms that her niece began to sing during her daily activities, such a rare occurrence that the whole family was dumbfounded, that she was happy as a lark.

To be sure of success and consolidate the cure I got the patient to come again from time to time, at greater intervals, and reiterated the same suggestions to her.

Over the course of the following years she occasionally came to rid herself of headaches. A single session most often sufficed. Her mood leaves nothing to be desired.

"All the anaemias which are not the result of a real organic disease, says Dr Wetterstrand[53], require treatment by hypnotic suggestion. Most of these patients are easily hypnotisable and most often reach a deep sleep. Louyet[54] even considers that anaemia constitutes the most sure indication of a disposition to enter the somnambulistic state." We are of the opinion that psycho-therapy is indicated above all in cases of anaemia which are superimposed on hysteria.

---

[53] Der Hypnotismus. S. 67. Wien 1891.

[54] Conf. Liébeault, Du sommeil et des états analogue. P. 451.

## OBS. 26

HYSTERICAL ANAEMIA, CHRONIC HEADACHES FOR FOUR YEARS, REFRACTORY TO MEDICAL TREATMENT, CURED BY PSYCHO-THERAPY.

Miss W. is chloro-anaemic[55]. She is 31 years old. She is only able to continue her occupation (as a piano teacher) with great difficulty, she has been so tormented in recent times by a chronic headache. Her doctor, after having treated her with drugs for almost four years, asked me to try psycho-therapy.

On the 16 Oct. 1892, Miss W. attended my clinic for the first time. She informed me that she had been ill for nearly four years. One evening, coming home tired from her lessons and going up stairs, she was completely overcome by piercing pulsations in her left ear. The sensation agitated and preoccupied her so much that she spent a sleepless night. Since that time she has slept badly; often she doesn't sleep at all, most of the time she only falls asleep towards the morning and has difficulty in waking up at her usual time (8am). The internal pulsation's perceptible in her ear come in fits and starts, and these episodes grow in frequency and end up being accompanied by a headache, finally degenerating into a very severe one. These headaches continue for about 24 hours but sometimes last for two or three days. Not a week goes by when she doesn't have at least one bout. She feels fatigued, mostly in her back and legs. This sensation of fatigue is greater in the first than the second half of the day.

---

[55] * Iron deficiency anaemia.

Pale mucosas. Her period is regular but the loss is insignificant, colourless and lasts less than 24 hours. Slow bowel movements. No appetite. Disgusted by meat, milk and eggs. She presents a hyperaesthetic zone on top of her head and is often affected by *globus*. Occasionally her throat feels constricted and painful for short periods of time, often she ends up suffering with heartburn. In summary, a hysterical anaemic suffering severe intractable headaches, refractory to medical and dietary treatment. I undertook treatment from the following day.

17 *Oct.* 1893. I obtain the charmed state[56] by suggestion. On awakening the patient assures me that the rest has done her good. I recommend that Miss W. feeds herself well and prescribe a diet that she has to follow rigorously. She should take meals regularly even, for example, when an attack of heartburn makes her not feel like eating. I promise her that thanks to daily treatment, my suggestions should rid her of her disgust for certain foods and of her pains, that gradually her nights will improve.

Every morning at the same time I carried out a session. The patient stayed somnolent for about an hour and received my suggestions. This treatment was punctiliously followed until the 21 February 1893. On that date a great improvement could be seen.

The patient had not been hearing the pulsations in her left ear for some time, the original symptom of her illness. Weeks had passed without a fit of headaches occurring. When a headache did occur, it

---

[56] Variety of somnambulism described by Dr Albert Pitres.

was not as intense as before and a simple suggestion on my part always sufficed to remove it.

There was no longer any disgust for food. She had a good appetite and often ate more than the prescribed rations. She ate two eggs, 1½ litres of milk and two large meals every day. The heartburn resisted my suggestions for longest. However recently she has not suffered with it. The fatigue in her leg and back has disappeared. Most of the time she sleeps well and all night long, it rarely takes her more than quarter of an hour to get off to sleep.

A stay of a few weeks in the country would certainly do her good, only she won't hear of it and continues to give her lessons. She is very happy with the results obtained and prefers life in town where she has her activities, to the possibility of the country putting some colour back in her cheeks. To consolidate the cure, which has been maintained, I gave her the occasional session until the end of May.

People subject to spontaneous somnambulism are principally hysterics. We had to treat two of these cases. In both cases we succeeded in plunging the patients into a deep sleep from the first session. Cure was obtained without difficulty.

**OBS. 27**

SPONTANEOUS SOMNAMBULISM, CURED BY ONE SESSION OF SUGGESTION.

A lay sister, aged 27 years, cares for an in-patient in my clinic. Although enjoying excellent health, she is affected by a symptom which is worrying for her patient, notably somnambulism. Having learnt that the nurse gets up from time to time during her sleep and goes about her business while sleeping, that she knows nothing of what she's done in that state when she wakes up, and that this merry-go-round agitates and worries her patient, I proposed to rid her of this undesirable habit by suggestion. Miss X. couldn't have wished for more. I find out that she was orphaned at the age of eight, she also has two brothers who are in good health.

She is unable to give me any information regarding her parents state of health nor their death. As for herself, she has never had a serious illness, however she did have the occasional headache, and sometimes broke alternately into spontaneous fits of laughter and tears, she is very impressionable and highly sympathetic to the pain and suffering of others. If her patient feels any kind of pain, she immediately feels the same pain in the corresponding place. Otherwise, she is a fine girl who valiantly carries out her duties. She has sometimes woken up in the middle of the night and found herself outside her bed packing her case in order to do something or other. This agitated and worried her, particularly the first time it happened.

28 *Dec.* 1890. One day, the nurse — during my visit to her patient — told me that she had a headache. I casually placed my hand on her forehead at which point she suddenly exclaimed: " Good God! Good God! How that comforts me, look my headache's gone. Thank you doctor."

Profiting from her extreme suggestibility and unbeknown to Miss X., I had succeeded in hypnotising her by surprise.

After having put the sick patient to sleep, I addressed myself to the nurse and affirmed that she would go into a deep sleep from the moment that her hand touched a certain object that I indicated. Laughing incredulously she touched the object with her finger and fell asleep instantaneously. Complete analgesia, pronounced catalepsy, realisation of various suggestions, in brief she was in a suggested state of deep somnambulism. She replies in a low voice to the questions I ask, enjoys her sleepy state and promises me she will never get up at night during her sleep. After ten minutes of profound sleep I bring her round. She is amazed, understands nothing of what has happened, complete amnesia.

During the following two months while Miss X was continuing to care for the patient in my clinic, she didn't experience a single episode of spontaneous somnambulism.

For some time gynaecologists have been more circumspect in their use of, and more scrupulous in their indications for mutilating operations. Only too often in the past, patients with hysterical and neurasthenic states, either manifest or latent, were misunderstood. On many occasions, once the operation was over, one had to recognise that the symptoms (pains, neuralgias, depression or excitement, paraesthesiae etc.) which had been attributed to local sepsis in an organ, were not slow in reappearing, be it immediately after the operation or some time later. Very often latent hysteria existing prior to the operation powerfully manifested itself afterwards.

We call to mind the observation of a colleague, a renowned practitioner who wanted to refer one of his patients to us who had become paraplegic and presented various indubitably hysterical symptoms following a third operation. For localised pains, he had successively first ablated one ovary, then the other, and finally carried out a hysterectomy. The patient furthermore, not having the least faith in the power of hypnotism, recused herself at the last minute and went to seek treatment elsewhere. The colleague *"swore, but a little late, that he would no longer take her on."*

## OBS. 28

OBSESSIVE EROTIC DREAMS, MENORRHAGIA. CURETTAGE OF THE WOMB. PERIODS BECOME NORMAL. NERVOUS SYMPTOMS PERSIST. BILATERAL OOPHORECTOMY. AGGRAVATION OF NERVOUS STATE. MARKED IMPROVEMENT THROUGH HYPNOTIC SUGGESTION.

*Family history.*

The patient's parents hadn't presented any nervous symptoms, the father is alive and enjoys good health, the mother died of a cancer. One of the patient's sisters died during an epileptic fit.

*Personal history.*

Mrs R. was a very nervous child, menarche at fourteen, she suffered from chest pains from her fifteenth to twentieth year, the date of her marriage. During the early years of her marriage her health was excellent notwithstanding six pregnancies at about yearly intervals. The illness began sometime after her penultimate confinement (July 1889). Her periods only returned three months later, they were heavy and irregular. Her psychological problems recurred. Insomnia, headaches, sensations of irritation, heaviness in her legs and in her lower abdomen, and in addition exhausting erotic dreams tormented the patient. A specialist called in by her family doctor advised curettage. That operation was followed by a reduction in blood loss and a new pregnancy (Dec. 1890). Its influence on the nervous system was negligible. Severe during the first half of her pregnancy, the nervous phenomena diminished in intensity and then completely disappeared during the second half, with the exception of the erotic dreams which increased in frequency occurring up to four times in a single night. Treatment with electricity brought some relief, a diminution of the dreams. In Sept. 1891 Mrs R. gave birth to an idiot child. After her confinement her sleep was adequate but she continued to be troubled by erotic dreams at night and her periods were irregular. A second consultation with a gynaecologist was followed by bilateral oophorectomy (March 1892).

It is true that the operation totally cured her menorrhagia, but its effect on her nervous symptoms was absolutely nil. Her insomnia returned, the patient refused to eat, she complained of congestion in her brain, pains in her limbs; sometimes her brain cleared and the erotic dreams tormented her unceasingly.

She consulted a professor in an inpatient clinic who advised her to try psycho-therapy.

Instead of following his advice she went to a charlatan, an unqualified doctor who, under the pretext that she was syphilitic, saturated her with potassium iodide and mercury. However her nervous condition got worse and worse, the patient weakened and finished by consulting her own doctor once again. She asked his opinion on a treatment by hypnotic suggestion.

The doctor was of the opinion that Mrs R. wouldn't make a good subject, that she wouldn't go to sleep. He advised her rather to undergo a clitoridectomy. Before deciding on this last option Mrs R. preferred to try hypnotic suggestion.

29 January 1893.

*Present state.* Small thin and slender woman, relates the vicissitudes of her history in a rambling manner. Of the different symptoms that torment her, the one she most fears is the erotic dream. She is even frightened of going to sleep because of the dream which pursues her to the point of obsession. The dream is always the same: her husband makes an advance, takes her, and the act is followed by a sensation of irritation in her lower abdomen especially her genitals accompanied by a serous secretion. She assures me that she doesn't experience the least voluptuous sensation but a feeling of enormous tiredness. The frequent production of serous secretions has produced an irritation of the cutaneous tissue on the upper and inside surfaces of her thighs.

At irregular intervals during the day, just as at night, the sensation described in her lower abdomen and private parts sometimes suddenly occurs; sometimes it is preceded by an analogous sensation in her head or occurs concurrently with it, without the dream or any lewd ideas.

She often has headaches. Her appetite has been lacking for a long time. She eats little and irregularly. Sometimes she feels like eating but as soon as she serves herself with something she is overtaken by disgust. Her bowel movements are retarded. The least exercise tires her out. She gets worked up over nothing. Moods changeable.

No other hysterical stigmata. On examination I note the presence of a scar on her abdomen, the absence of ovaries, and I find the skin of her thighs lightly scratched. No hyperexcitability of the abdomen or clitoris.

I began treatment on the same day. From the first sessions the patient showed herself to be very amenable to suggestion. I gave an appointment every day at the same time and obtained a deep sleep. The patient gradually regained calm sleep, and the dreams diminished in frequency, her appetite returned and the patient recovered her strength and good humour, her bowels moved regularly each morning. By the second half of April 1893 the patient's condition was so much improved that her husband assured me he couldn't remember ever having seen his wife so happy and well disposed.

She had no sexual appetite, she submitted passively to her husband's advances — in any case very rare. However the accomplishment of the act was always followed by a sleepless night.

The 1 May following, Mrs R. left Amsterdam for a town in the provinces. She continued to see me twice a week. At first everything went well. However the very hot summer's days affected the patient badly and made her journey (½ hour by train) unbearable. The fatigue of the journey often caused her a bad night. So I provisionally advised Mrs R. to discontinue the treatment until Autumn.

1 Dec. 1893. Mr R. came to give me news of his lady, which was good regarding her dreams which no longer obsessed her and only occurred rarely. On the other hand there were still complaints. She was capricious and complained of irregular sleep, all exercise tired her out, and the piano which she used to very much love playing,

now annoyed her. She dared not come by train to see me in Amsterdam because she knew the journey would cost her sleep on the following night. From time to time she complained of heart palpitations and chest pain.

I advised Mr R. to come back to live in Amsterdam where he had his business, so that his wife could receive my care from time to time when she felt the need.

The following observation falls within the category of nosophobia[57] that one mainly encounters in neurasthenics but which affects hysterics just as much.

## OBS. 29

HAEMOPTYSIS APPARENTLY HYSTERICAL, RESISTANT TO MEDICAL TREATMENT, CURED BY HYPNOTIC SUGGESTION.

A young person, sister of one of my patients suffering from hystero-epileptic fits, was referred to me on 5 Dec. 1892 by her doctor.

There are many nervous members of her family. She too has often presented a range of hysterical symptoms: nervous fits, globus, bouts of laughing and crying. For some months she has occasionally spat blood, sometimes spontaneously without coughing, mainly associated with some kind of emotion, sometimes after making an effort to cough.

---

[57] * Fear of having a specific disease.

It is true the quantity of blood is always minimal. It is often only slightly coloured mucous infiltrated with blood that she brings up; however the symptom worries the patient to a very high degree. She is afraid that her lungs may be involved and that she may be phthisic. Repeated examination by her doctor, a most conscientious man, has been unable to appease her fears since his medicine remains ineffective.

On examination I found absolutely nothing to be worried about, her respiratory organs, heart and stomach showed no objective pathology. Inspection of her mouth, nose and throat revealed nothing abnormal.

Although slim, Miss L. is well built, her thorax is well formed, adipose tissue sufficiently developed.

There is a slight hardening of the ear following a sclerosis of the tympanic cavities and a catarrh of the Eustachian tubes.

No appetite. Sensation of heaviness in the stomach. Retarded bowel movements. Globus. Sleep is agitated, troubled by dreams. On waking the patient coughs a lot and brings up bloody sputum.

The patient is compliant to the suggestion of sleep. Profound hypnosis. However the principal phenomenon only gradually disappeared after several weeks treatment. It was only after three months that a cure was obtained.

If it is conceded that during profound sleep and enhanced suggestibility, functional troubles are more easily corrected than in a waking state or light sleep, it must also be recognised that in spite of obtaining the state favouring cure, it can be a long time in coming. Thus, in the following observation the phenomenon of "drying up" stimulated by obsessive emotion, although suppressed by suggestion in a state of somnambulism, was not slow in recurring sooner or later after every session. It was also necessary to redo, so to speak, the singing education of the patient during and after each sleep, in order to definitively destroy her obsessional idea.

## OBS. 30.

ANXIETY STATE, CAUSING INABILITY TO SING AND LACK OF EFFORT TO MEMORISE IN A HYSTERIC, PUPIL OF THE CONSERVATOIRE, CURED BY HYPNOTIC SUGGESTION.

Miss N. is 28 years old. She has attended the music conservatoire for four years, possesses a beautiful voice and thanks to her talent and application was expected to pursue a fine career. However she is very nervous. Above all during recent months her agitation has rendered her unable to get a note out in front of her masters, while when alone or with friends she's completely in possession of her voice and sings very well. The presence of her teachers or of a public causes her so much anxiety that she ceases to think, is unable to reply to the most simple question put to her, and finds it literally impossible to sing. Should this state of affairs persist, she would be forced to abandon her studies and say good-bye to a career that was beckoning her and that she would have embraced with dedication.

Her parents, not very well off, had suffered privations in order to allow her to pursue her studies; also Miss N. finds herself doubly unhappy, first because of her nervous state which makes it impossible for her to pass her examination, and then because she sees herself as never being able to pay them back. She no longer sleeps at night, refuses to eat and is falling into a state of extreme psychological depression.

On 15 April 1891, having heard speak of cures for nervous states obtained by hypnotism, she came to consult me and ask my advice.

*Family history.*

Father and mother hysterics. Of twelve brothers and sisters only three are exempt from functional nervous problems. The maternal grandmother was a grand hysteric.

*Personal history.*

Miss N. never presented nervous troubles characteristic of hysteria other than abrupt changes of mood for no apparent reason, whims, a capricious appetite, a habit of talking in her sleep and various fears. Never had a illness.

*Present state.* No hysterical stigmata. With tears in her eyes and in a desperate tone of voice, Miss N., who otherwise seemed well and much younger than her age, recounted her troubles. After a thorough examination which reveals the absolute absence of organic lesions, I reassure the patient and promise to cure her.

An initial session given the following day did her a lot of good. She went to sleep by suggestion and felt momentarily relieved of her obsessive anxiety.

I repeat the sessions every day and concentrate at first on giving her a good night's sleep and getting her back into a balanced frame of mind. The hypnotic sleep gradually deepens and after several sessions I obtain profound somnambulism. I make use of it to get her to do singing exercises and suggest that she is singing in front of her teacher or a real audience. I get her to repeat her lessons and prove to her that her memory isn't at fault from the moment she allows herself not to be obsessed by anxiety. Later these exercises were continued not only in a sleeping state but also in a waking state in the presence of several people, friends at first, then strangers.

And so I gained some ground and slowly she recovered her confidence. I advised her to repeat her last year, which she did. After a treatment of fourteen months the patient passed her examination with honours and felt relieved of her anxiety. This result was acquired through patience and perseverance. There were many occasions when partial setbacks alternated with periods of progress, especially during the early months. I always succeeded in lifting her spirits, giving her encouragement and strengthening her determination to go on.

The high level of suggestibility which she exhibited in the somnambulistic state provided a precious tool for establishing auto-suggestions in the patient and for neutralising some hysterical symptoms such as mutism, inability to open the eyes, pains, fits of tears and laughter etc.

I always succeeded easily in preventing latent hysteria from gaining power.

After obtaining her diploma she was able to take part in an artistic tour of Europe and on her return, her singing and piano teacher offered her a place in a young women's music school. A place which she accepted and fulfilled with honour from then until now (August 1894).

Occasionally during vacations Miss N. comes to see me, and between times the exchange of letters provides me with the opportunity to give her advice. Little by little her self-confidence is growing and soon she should be able to completely dispense with my psychological support.

The results we obtained by psychological treatment of neurasthenia and neurasthenic conditions lead us to believe that psycho-therapy is the treatment of choice for this neurosis. The majority of patients that we treated only had recourse to us after having tried the various usual medical approaches.

Now a therapy which under these circumstances can produce a notable improvement in 35 cases and a cure in 21 cases out of 99 under treatment, has every right to its place in the sun. There is a need for it.

In his book "Hypnotisme , Suggestion, Psycho-therapie", Professor Bernheim sums up his views on hereditary neurasthenia thus:

"When neurasthenia is hereditary, when it is due to an inborn malconfiguration of the nervous system, then one must have the courage to say that most often it is incurable. The patients are sometimes difficult to hypnotise, their brain is obsessed by so many impressions or such tenacious ones, psychological, sensory and visceral, that it often resists all suggestion. Despite their complicity, their goodwill, their desire to let themselves be hypnotised and to get better, their nervous system can offer an invincible resistance to all attempts at influencing it. There are some who are responsive to hypnotism, however although they fall into a profound sleep, they are not always compliant with therapeutic suggestions. Sometimes one is able to momentarily calm their symptoms, one removes their pain and various nervous troubles: there is a notable improvement, one hopes for a more or less complete cure. That improvement can be lasting, sustained by prolonged or repeated suggestion. That's a lot! With others the cure is only temporary. Soon auto-suggestion retakes the whole of its empire, the illness reappears in all its intensity, the patients and the doctor lose confidence in suggestive treatment, the poor unfortunates run from one specialist to another, soak their miseries in all the mineral waters, go from hydrotherapy to massage, from homeopathy to dosimetry or Mattei's granules[58]. Sometimes an improvement occurs under the influence of one of these treatments; a remission more or less long asserts itself, *post hoc* or *propter hoc*, followed by a relapse! That's the sad odyssey of numerous neuropaths due to the fatal law of heredity! The only thing I note, alas! is that when suggestion is impotent, so is everything else."

From our point of view, no neurasthenic is *per se* incurable. However the cure of these patients by psychotherapy requires the creation of particular conditions adapted to the individual needs of each case. Alas in too many cases various circumstances prevent the patient from pursuing such a treatment!

Psychotherapy clinics should be set up to begin with in large centres where a sufficient population of neurotics can

---

[58] treatment based on homeopathic-like *granules* enhanced with vegetable electricity that *Mattei* believed could restore the balance between body electric charges.

be found. Rather than disposing of neurasthenics or hysterics by getting them to travel, sending them to the waters, stuffing them with bromides and, so to speak, multiple anti-nervous preparations, we could choose an appropriate milieu for them in the same town, or if there is nothing against it we could let them stay in their own home. For the majority of these patients intellectual or manual work according to their psychological or physical capacity is essential and where better to find it than in their own place of residence? The main thing for these patients is to find in their doctor a person in whom they can in all conscience rely, who knows how to understand and guide them.

In treatment thus understood, suggestion plays an outstanding role. At first one will mainly have recourse to frequent and prolonged sessions. If on the one hand neurasthenics are good sleepers, on the other many have lost the habit of regular sleep. These patients need to relearn to sleep; one accustoms them to lying down and resting tranquilly for part of a day at the same time, with eyes closed, listening to suggestions of calm and wellbeing that the doctor repeats from time to time, suggestions that they will then ruminate on and gradually put into practice.

Although the doctor has an easier task with good sleepers, in so far as he can dispense with the re-education of this function, one shouldn't think that by this fact alone he can triumph with the greatest of ease over other morbid symptoms. Even the deep sleeper, the somnambulist, doesn't always respond to therapeutic suggestion. Both with the sleeper and the patient who fails to sleep, one has to be able to reason, to know how to find the weak point and to operate at the right physiological moment, in order to allow an idea to be introduced and accepted. From the beginning of treatment one has to instil in the patient the need to be satisfied with a more or less considerable improvement in their state. They have to understand that a congenitally nervous constitution inevitably makes them vulnerable to relapses and that their organs are not at fault, rather in their case it is a question of an imbalance of forces. A thorough examination, repeated from time to time, will serve to both reassure the patient and prevent the doctor from following a false path and misconstruing the nature of the symptoms: an organic illness can be superimposed on a functional nervous syndrome or come to light during the course treatment. One cannot repeat often enough that the presenting phenomena are the expression of functional troubles arising from a psychological or somatic shock and maintained or nourished by the patient's imagination.

A weakness of will, a lack of confidence in their own strength, a fear of having a dangerous or incurable illness has been installed in their brain, acting as an auto-suggestion contrary and opposed to the disappearance of their symptoms.

The role, the duty of the doctor practicing psycho-therapy, involves winning the confidence of the patient to a very high degree, serving him as both a friend and guide. Armed with these qualities he will know how to lift the morale of the patient in moments of weakness and apathy, insist on an effort of will, get him to continue methodical exercise, train him, harden him, encourage him by reiterating the progress he has made. He will relieve him of undue anxiety and possible discouragement, predicting that a relapse might happen, but saying that they are to a certain extent characteristic and normal in neurotic conditions, and will occur less and less frequently and become less severe if the patient continues to do his best to follow exactly the prescribed regime. Then when there is a clear indication of improvement, the doctor will teach him to gradually relinquish the moral support of his suggestions and replace it with appropriate auto-suggestions, all the time giving the patient to understand that he will always find his doctor ready to help if the need arises, be it in order to prevent a relapse, or to put him back on the right track if his equilibrium has become disturbed.

Envisaged this way, the treatment of neurasthenia is, so to speak, a perpetual cure, but it is the only rational one and leads infallibly to the goal. It doesn't make a slave out of the patient but a friend. In this sense alone one can speak of carrying out the cure of hysterics and neurasthenics. We are convinced that the future of treatment for these neuroses is by psycho-therapy understood in this way.

**OBS. 31.**

CEREBRAL NEURASTHENIA. HEADACHES. INABILITY TO CONTINUE HIS STUDIES IN A STUDENT. CURE.

A medical student aged 20 years, counted several neurasthenics and melancholics among the members his family, a paternal uncle committed suicide. His father, who had died several years before, was neurasthenic.

He came to me on the 14 May 1888 for a severe headache which prevented him from studying. Registered as a student in 1882, he had studied with enthusiasm and taken his first examinations, which conferred the title of Candidate in Medicine on him in Dec. 1885. Since then, however, despite his best efforts, he had been unable to continue his studies. All reading tired him out and disturbed him. If he tried to read a page he didn't take in a word, when he got to the bottom of the page he knew just about as much as when he began to read. If he tried to make himself re-read the passage, the lines, the words, the letters got all mixed up and he felt a sensation of tension, heaviness in his head followed by a headache. Cerebral fatigue also occurred when he conversed, above all when the subject required some effort of thought.

He followed his professors' courses assiduously and gained a lot from them, especially certain subjects in which he was particularly interested. Other than that, he scarcely did anything but hang about. He went to bed late, slept very well and found it difficult to get out of bed in the morning. He felt most tired during the mornings, it was also during that part of the day that he had his headaches. He experienced them as a sense of constriction in his forehead, temporal fossae, in the occipital region and on the top of his head. After lunch the headaches diminished and they disappeared in the afternoon. He felt most well in the evenings.

*Present state.* A young man of medium height, well built, looking nothing less than ill. Slight myopia corrected by glasses. Small scar on forehead. Is a little agitated when I examine and question him. He is in the throws of a headache at the time, he describes it as feeling as if the skin on his forehead and top of his head was stuck to the epicranial aponeurosis. Excellent appetite. Bowels open regularly. Takes no exercise, no venereal disease, no alcohol, leads a very organised life. Often has heart palpitations, a raised pulse of 90 on average. On examination, nothing abnormal regarding his heart. He despairs of ever finishing his doctorate, since study is impossible for him. He supposes that suggestion might be of benefit, however he fears he may not be sufficiently suggestible. He bases this opinion on the fact that he turned up on the scene when Donato[59] was in Amsterdam, and found himself unmoved.

An initial attempt at hypnotism immediately succeeded; a little agitation at first, a nervous laugh avoiding eye contact with me, then a marked drowsiness as soon as I closed his eyelids. After a half hour's sleep I woke up the young man who found that his headache had gone.

I advised the patient to come and see me every day, to provisionally abstain from all reading, but to continue to follow assiduously the oral and clinical teaching of his masters and to prepare himself in this way for his doctoral examination. After a month of treatment, it was already possible for him to read for half an hour without feeling any untoward sensations. The deep hypnotic sleep in which I plunged him in my daily sessions promoted the putting into practice of my suggestions: the disappearance of the helmet sensation, the reestablishment of the ability to read without getting tired. During the summer vacation he was already able to allow himself two or three hours of intense study and on the 2 Oct. 1888 he took the first part of his doctoral examination with success. Having obtained this first success, his progress was enhanced. In March 1889 he took the second part of his doctorate, and finally in Oct. 1889 the title of Doctor of Medicine was conferred on him. After his success in the first test,

---

[59] *Donato, a stage hypnotist.

the sessions were spaced out more and more. From time to time the headaches returned but always disappeared under the influence of an appropriate suggestion.

In March 1890 I saw my patient for the last time, he was cheerful, in good spirits, very well and completely happy. He left the country in order to go to the colonies in the Indies where he had been appointed to a medical officer's post.

## OBS. 32.

NEURASTHENIC SYMPTOMS CURED BY HYPNOTIC SUGGESTION.

A young provincial doctor, 33 years of age, robust constitution, healthy looking, asked me to rid him, if possible, of certain neurasthenic symptoms which were sometimes bothersome.

He lost his father when he was 5 years old, who died from cancer of the stomach and liver. His mother was a very nervous woman who had suffered much unhappiness in her life, above all as a result of the bad behaviour of two of her sons who were addicted to drink, one of whom had recently died. The patient had a sister troubled by sciatica.

From an early age Doctor X suffered from depression and bouts of melancholia, he had always been very irritable. For a long time he believed that he had to attribute his nervous condition to family problems, however, since he began to study medicine he decided he was suffering from neurasthenia. In contrast to the harmful predilections of his brothers, the patient exhibits an exemplary sobriety. He established a medical practice 5 years ago and married the following year. He is happily married, enjoys a good reputation as a doctor and has an excellent clientele.

*Present state* 18 Nov. 1892.

For some months the patient has suffered from a heaviness and sense of compression of his head by a band stretching from his forehead along his temples to the occipital region. This sensation makes him morose, indifferent to everything, unable to do his work. He finds it difficult to give the desired attention to his patients' complaints. The sensation, however, is not permanent. Most often he has his headaches in the mornings. He feels tiredness in his legs and pains in the coccygeal region. He goes to bed late often staying awake till the early hours of the morning. In the mornings he is tired and finds it difficult to get out of bed. His stomach is temperamental, symptoms of dyspepsia. Coinciding with the sensation of heaviness in his head he passes water infrequently. As soon as the diuresis increases the heaviness in his head disappears. Some time ago he abandoned his practice for a fortnight and spent holidays with a colleague to try and get himself together. This break didn't do him any good. With the exception of potassium bromide which he prescribes for himself from time to time, he abstains from all medication.

Dr X found himself to be very amenable to suggestion. I succeeded in inducing a deep sleep from the first session. He was able to continue with his work. I treated him with hypnotic suggestion from 18 Nov. 1892 to the end of March 1893, with resounding success. He came to see me firstly three times then twice and finally once a week. All his symptoms have disappeared and now (January 1894) he continues to enjoy excellent health.

## OBS. 33.

SEVERE NEURASTHENIA, DATING BACK TEN YEARS, REFRACTORY TO ALL TREATMENT. NOTABLE AND PERSISTENT IMPROVEMENT THANKS TO TREATMENT BY SUGGESTION CONTINUED AND LASTING MORE THAN 4 YEARS.

*Family history.*

A nervous family. The father, a man coming up to his 80th year was always very irritable, irascible, but nonetheless enjoyed good health. The mother tends toward melancholy, is constantly preoccupied with her health, is always looking for care. One brother is a hereditary neurasthenic. Another brother is subject to uncontrollable headaches.

*Personal history.*

Born in 1850, the patient had no serious illnesses in his childhood. He lived a measured life, sometimes masturbated, never to excess. Intern in a business enterprise, he was noted for his ambition and application, succeeded in this trade and ended up by marrying the daughter and becoming the partner of his boss. (Oct. 1879).

Three months after the consummation of the marriage, the patient was afflicted by nervous episodes which very soon developed into the complete syndrome of severe neurasthenia. During the following years, Mr X. followed the usual treatments and lived abroad for a long time without gaining the least benefit in the world, ending up with an absolute disbelief in doctors and medicines. He withdrew from business, hid himself away somewhere in the country and has already abstained from all treatment for more than a year. Before this despair hit him he had been advised to try psycho-therapy but he wouldn't hear of it. However, in early October 1889 hearing of the miraculous cure by hypnotism of a man known to him, who had been suffering for a long time from a nervous illness very similar to his own, he decided to come to see me.

*Present state.* On 18 Oct. 1889 Mr. X. accompanied by his brother-in-law was brought by carriage to my clinic. He is a strong, well built man, 38 years of age, he appears healthy, his face is ruddy; however his eyes are dull, his limbs dangle, and there is a general impression of tiredness, unhappiness and dejection. He tells me the history of his illness in a slow, disconnected way, indicative of a severe psychological condition that contrasts with his physique.

The patient complains of prolonged irregular but frequent bouts of migraine. A sensation of dull pressure in his occipital region, irritating febrile heat in his forehead and at the top of his head disturbing him incessantly. Bright light irritates him and all reading tires him out.

He has continuous pains in his kidneys and a sensation of heaviness and tiredness forces him to remain with his back bent forward whilst in a sitting position. His favourite position where he suffers the least, is lying horizontally flat.

He can walk and carry out all movements requested, but he moves as little as possible because all movement increases his pains. He feels tired all the time, even the effort of thinking makes him tired. Complete inertia and apathy paralyses him in everything. He often cries, he has crazy fears, triggered by what he reads in the papers, by stories of illnesses or poverty. His animal life doesn't suffer. He eats well, digests perfectly, he is a good sleeper, gets up late in the morning. From time to time however, bouts of of precordial anxiety[60] and heart palpitations give rise to sleepless nights and heighten his miseries. His sexual appetite is moderate. Bowels move regularly.

On the front of his thorax and abdomen there is an enormous chloasma[61], almost as large as the palms of two hands. No worrying lesions found on examination, I gave Mr. X. to understand that he could be cured without any doubt if he would give me his confidence and have a meaningful and prolonged trial of treatment by suggestion.

I gave him his first session on the same day and succeeded in putting him to sleep and giving him a feeling of well-being. He woke up relieved. I continued the treatment every day at the same time. At the end of the first week, Mr. X. cancelled the carriage and from then on made the trip from his house to my clinic (a distance

---

[60] Intense beating of the heart accompanied by anxiety and shortness of breath.

[61] *Patch of grey-brown pigmentation.

of half an hour) by tram. At the end of the first month, he was in a state where he could take a half-hour walk and give a business consultation to a client. The improvement continued until 1 Dec. 1889. On that date, the first relapse. Return of all his symptoms, with the exception of the migraine. Enormous psychological depression. However, he continued with the cure. My sessions relieved him, but the symptoms returned almost immediately afterwards. From the 11 December his condition improved, the patient began to use the tram again, which he had abandoned in favour of a carriage. With periods alternately better and worse we managed to get to the 30 July 1891. At that time he was he was able to stand in for his business partner for a fortnight. From then on he attended the office every day and gradually began to participate in running the daily business. He went from strength to strength. During December 1891 the daily sessions were interrupted by an intercurrent illness, notably influenza, which Mr. X. survived perfectly well without any exacerbation of neurasthenic symptoms. From April 1892 he was able to take over the direction of his business completely and to cope with the exigencies of social life, making and receiving visits etc.

In August 1892, after a vacation of one month that I had agreed to, I found Mr. X. in the midst of a relapse. He was depressed, broken down, had an irrational fear of cholera and wasn't sleeping at night. However several sessions staved off the enemy and got the patient back on his feet. From February 1893, Mr. X's condition was so satisfactory that I was able to reduce the suggestive sessions to three times a week.

During the course of the treatment the patient had only had two attacks of migraine. He goes for at least a two hour walk every day without getting tired, he reads a lot, deals perfectly with his business affairs, no longer suffers at all with his eyes, he is cheerful, fit and well and one couldn't be more satisfied with his condition.

I am continuing with his treatment.

## OBS. 34.

SEVERE NEURASTHENIA; NOTABLE IMPROVEMENT. RELAPSE.

On the 14 August 1890, I received a visit from a retired Royal Nederland's Navy doctor, who asked me if I would treat him for neurasthenic problems.

*Family history.*

His father is a neuropath, his mother had been admitted several times to a nursing home and treated for hysterical mania. One of his sisters is a hysteric who has a range of symptoms.

*Personal history.*

Due to his mother's mental condition, the patient was brought up by his grandparents in a provincial town. He was constantly in the company of older people, he rarely had the occasion to play with children of is own age. This resulted in a precocious knowledge of things and people that it is better for a child to be unaware of.

Although he was very much loved, he was not a happy child. He doesn't remember having had any serious childhood illnesses.

He did very well in primary school and then at the lycée and became a medical student at the University of Amsterdam at the age of 19. From his 14th year, he developed the habit of masturbating and became passionately attached to this vice. The beginning of his nervous trouble dates from that time, manifesting itself in alternate bouts of melancholy and exuberant gaiety.

He applied himself seriously to his studies, but this cost him a lot of effort. He gave up his bad habit and visited a prostitute from time to time. At that time he was already suffering from a nervous inadequacy; ejaculation during the coital act taking place prematurely, before or immediately after the introduction of the virile member.

He took all his examinations on time and acquitted himself well. Among comrades, he was considered to be very knowledgeable and to have a great facility for learning. According to him, nothing could have been further from the truth, he had to struggle and spend sleepless nights in order to succeed.

Appointed doctor at the age of 26, he received his nomination as a military medical officer in the Royal Nederland's Navy.

Life on board, his time in the tropics, the whole new world which unfolded in front of his eyes, left him with happy, pleasant associations. He remembers this period of his life with great pleasure. However, none the less, he was often unhappy, irritable and troubled by a tiredness of his whole being, a fatigue that he just couldn't explain to himself. He slept badly and tried to get some sleep with the help of alcoholic drinks, which incidentally he hated. He didn't exceed certain limits and preferred to be awake all night rather than run the risk of getting drunk. He never had recourse to narcotics, fearing addiction to morphine. He often had bouts of precordial pain and suicidal ideas.

Good and bad phases alternated. He carried out his duties well and was respected as a doctor, well liked by his comrades. Being ambitious, the idea of not being able to read and study at his leisure without having to put up with mental fatigue which forced him to put down his book, distressed him.

After four years service in the Indian archipelago he served two years at Leyde in navigation school, then returned to the Indies on board a frigate.

During this voyage, in a fit of psychological depression, resolving to end his life, he let himself fall down a flight of twenty stairs. He was left with some bruises but found himself relieved of his melancholy for some time. Several months later in the Bay of Batavia, sad ideas took hold of him again, he was admitted to hospital, provisionally sorted out and sent back to Europe.

On arrival in Holland, he was granted unlimited leave. He used it to consult several foreign medical authorities, such as Professors Erb and Rosenthal. He spent some time in Vienna where he underwent electrotherapy then returned to Holland in order to take a ten month hydrotherapy cure. After these cures he was just as sick as before, the Naval Medical Commission definitively reassessed him and he was retired on grounds of nervous ill health following on from brain concussion, arising from an accident on board during service.

Having left the service, my colleague first had a feeling of relaxation. He felt relieved of medical responsibility which had weighed very heavily upon him during his last days in the Navy. However this state of quietude didn't last long. Returning to the paternal home he soon found himself just as unhappy as he was before. He became sad, morose, stopped sleeping, refused the narcotics that his father (a pharmacist) urged him to take. He accused himself of having cheated the authorities by hiding the fact that he had deliberately let himself fall down the stairs, so that the retirement pension he had been given was actually a theft he had committed from the state etc.

A suicide attempt by hanging was noticed in time and prevented. A passing calm followed this period of excitement. Several days afterwards, at the recommendation of the Naval Inspector of Healthcare who had been to see him, he came to consult me and asked me to look after him.

*Present state 14 august 1890.*

Nervous man, agitated, average constitution, complaining of precordial anxiety, worries, aboulia[62], incessant doubt. He is particularly preoccupied by and ruminates over this question: did I have an accidental fall on board or did I intentionally let myself fall meaning to kill myself. If the latter is correct, I am a thief and

---

[62] *Lack of motivation.

haven't the right to touch one centime of the retirement pension given to me.

He complains of heart palpitations and insomnia. He often used to drink beer and cognac in the evenings in order to sleep. However he has ceased drinking for fear of becoming drunk. Occasionally he has taken bromides never for a long time and always in small doses. He has often made use of chloral hydrate and sulfonyl, never morphine for fear of becoming addicted.

He is tired all the time, however it doesn't stop him shopping for several hours; in the evenings he feels most at ease. He talks a lot, never stops moving, couldn't remain seated for a quarter of an hour.

He can't seriously concentrate on anything. He can't read, that is to say when he tries to read his thoughts are elsewhere, furthermore reading tires him out and gives him headaches.

Appetite excellent. He eats a lot. Always feels a bit better after a good meal. No digestive troubles. Bowels normal. On examination no organic lesion.

He asks me to take him on as patient having put all his hope in a cure by suggestion.

From 14 August 1890 till 12 April 1891, I looked after the patient in my house as a member of the family. During this time he abstained completely from all medication and, with the exception of a glass of beer at table, from all alcoholic drink. My treatment had been simple suggestion. I was never able to obtain the least degree of sleep. He presented himself every day at the same time in my clinic, lay down on a chaise long, closed his eyes and stayed like that for one or two hours. During that time I placed myself near to him 3 or 4 times and made various suggestions according to his current symptoms. At first the effort required to remain calm and lying down cost him a great deal, however gradually he got used to it, then the habit became pleasant and agreeable. Soon he arrived early and greedily drank up, so to speak, my suggestions of calm and repose. He often got me to make very special ones for him or to repeat particular ones.

After some weeks, the irregular sleep began to get better, the anxiety calmed down, the patient took part in various family games (tric-trac, draughts, dominoes), got involved in making cardboard cut-outs. From the beginning of December his folie de doute, anxiety and melancholy disappeared and his sleep left nothing to be desired. He took up his favourite theoretical studies, skin diseases, at first studying for one hour per day, then little by little I pressured him into visiting the dermatological polyclinic. Soon he was attending it every day between 2 and 3 o'clock and playing an important role in treating the patients. From then on his morale went from strength to strength, he felt reborn, began to have faith in his abilities once again and recovered his identity as a doctor.

His irritable mood softened noticeably, he became agreeable, chatted and felt more and more at his ease.

During January, February and March, he made some visits to the paternal home, sometimes spending one or two nights there. In the end everything went well.

The cure was so well established that he thought seriously of setting up a specialist dermatological practice in Amsterdam.

However before establishing himself, which he proposed to do in Autumn 1891, he wanted to spend the summer in Paris in order to profit from the teaching of French experts. It was with this in mind that he left me for Paris on 12 April.

On that date he was perfectly well balanced. He left me a beautiful painting as a souvenir which he accompanied with these words:

"As witness to my gratitude and recognition of my cure and at the same time as a souvenir of my friendship."

My patient stayed in Paris from the 13 April to the 27 May 1891.

His early news dating from the 14 April was excellent. Then I heard nothing from him until the 9th of the following May. He wrote to me thus: "After scarcely more than a few days in the hell-fire of this great Paris, insomnia took hold of me, soon the precordial anxiety was added to it followed immediately by my preoccupations, my doubts, my melancholy."

On the 26th of the same month I went to Paris and found him in a state of over excitation such that I prevailed on him to return with me immediately to Amsterdam.

The contrast between the family life which he had led for several months — a regular life backed up by moderate exercise of body and mind, recreation according to his mood — with the chaotic life in the chasm of Paris where he found himself isolated, lacking moral support, where nobody gave a damn about him, proved to be too great. It is true that during the last month of his stay with me he was unaccustomed to have his suggestive sessions, but nevertheless he felt that I was there, that he only had to say something in order to get advice or an encouraging word.

The relapse was one of the most severe.

My suggestions no longer had the effect they used to have. The patient no longer completely opened himself up to me as before. After only three weeks of his renewed sojourn under my roof, he confessed to me the new cause of his obsessional preoccupations: he had become enamoured of one of the maids and although nothing serious had happened between himself and the girl before his departure for Paris, on arriving there he felt overcome by remorse, firstly with regard to the maid whom he had promised to take as a housewife as soon as he was set up as a specialist, then vis à vis myself because he had been the cause of impropriety under the roof of a friend and benefactor. Now he could no longer dream of getting set up, nor could he ever fulfil his promise to the maid etc. etc.

He asked me to sort out this business, to give presents. Far from being relieved after his confession, he was tormented by doubt: did I do something improper in my relations with the maid, yes or no? Sleep irregular. Anxiety. Thoughts of suicide. I seriously thought of transferring him into a nursing home, when after dinner on the 29th June while I was out, he was able to get hold of (being a doctor) an aqueous solution of 1 gramme chlorhydrate of morphine from a local pharmacist. It seemed that he immediately withdrew into his bedroom and swallowed the contents of the phial in one go.

Five hours later, on returning, I found him in a deep state of narcosis. All my efforts to save him came to nothing, he died on the 1st July at 7 o'clock in the morning.

## OBS. 35.

NEURASTHENIA. MOTOR ASTHENIA PREDOMINANT. NOTABLE IMPROVEMENT.

A neurasthenic lady had been treated for a long time with drugs, electricity and massage. She had been under the care of renowned specialists. She finally submitted herself to treatment by hypnotism. A doctor tried to hypnotise her but didn't succeed in getting her to sleep. Having failed to benefit from any of her treatments she decided to request my care.

*Present state* 9 Oct. 1888.

Miss V. is 24 years old, she is girlish. Her mother is a very nervous woman who often suffers from renal colic. Her father died a long time ago from heart disease. Of six brothers and sisters, one sister is a hysteric. She has never been seriously ill, but she has been troubled by facial acne since her earliest years. Her periods began in her 15th year, always irregular, most often they are late by 2 or 3 weeks, last for 4 days, are never heavy and always preceded by pains and followed by a milky secretion.[63]

---

[63] • *"fleurs blanches"*.

A small embonpoint, pale face and mucosas. Pulse 78 to 82, rather weak, the patient often has palpitations. She eats little, has no appetite, is in horror of meat, eggs and milk. Bowels regular. She sleeps badly, dreams a lot and often wakes in a start. Tired in the mornings, she feels better during the second half of the day and likes to go to bed late.

She suffers a good deal from headaches, characterised by a tightness in her forehead, temples and occipital region. Movement of her head often causes a cracking sensation in her neck. She is tired all the time and suffers from back pain radiating from her shoulders to her kidneys. She is so tired that she imagines she is unable to walk. Without doubt she can walk, however the effort is painful to her and costs her so much that she prefers not to move. When she does walk it gets worse. Her tendon reflexes are normal. Her reaction to faradic current is also normal. Muscular tremors in her thighs, hands and face. The dynamometer shows 27 Kg. for the right hand and 25 Kg. for the left hand. No sensory problems. Neither heart, generative organs nor any other organs show anatomical changes. The patient feels unable to walk more than 5 or 6 minutes at a time.

She kills time by doing handwork or lying on a sofa. She reads little because reading causes irritation in her eyes and tiredness.

A first attempt at hypnotising Miss V. succeeded pretty well. She became somnolent and compared the sensation she felt while in that stage to a light morphinic intoxication. A regular treatment with hypnotic suggestion was continued from that day until the end of June 1889. She was then free of headache, ate with appetite and had lost her excessive pallor. Her strength was so very much increased that the dynamometer showed 63 Kg. for the right hand and 58 Kg. for the left hand, and the patient was able to take a walk for two hours continuously every day without getting tired. She continued the sessions for about a year spaced at greater intervals to consolidate the cure. Since then she has left Amsterdam and gone abroad. The latest news dating from Sept. 1892 reports a relapse of her motor asthenia.

## OBS. 36.

SEVERE NEURASTHENIA. MOTOR ASTHENIA PREDOMINANT. NOTABLE AND PERSISTENT IMPROVEMENT OF THE PRINCIPAL PHENOMENA.

Young woman aged 20, comes under my care for a paralysis of her lower limbs which has lasted several months.

*Family history.*

The phthisic father died five years ago in a lunatic asylum. The mother is healthy, an energetic woman. Two of the patient's brothers died at a young age, one sister, older by a year, enjoys good health although she isn't robust.

Several members of the family, as much on the paternal as the maternal side, have nervous illnesses, some are insane.

*Personal history.*

As a child, she presented the symptoms of chronic hydrocephalus. From the age of 12 she suffered from prolonged weakness of her legs, with alternating periods of improvement and deterioration. She was often unable to stand up and walk for weeks and even months.

*Present state* 28 March 1892.

A debilitated young woman, anaemic, spends her days lying on a chaise longue. For six months she has been unable to walk. She stays on the chaise long all day and then in the evening leaves it for her bed. She suffers from severe headache at least five days in the week. If the pain isn't in her head it moves to her legs. She suffers continually from rachialgia[64] and tiredness in her back and limbs. Her hands are not just moist but always covered in sweat. All reading fatigues her. She can't even bear someone reading to her. Any handwork such as sewing or knitting causes her pain and increases her sense of weakness.

No appetite, she always feeds herself with three beaten eggs mixed with a litre of milk per day. Bowels normal. Menstruation regular, however the loss is minimal. Often complains of hyperaesthesia of the scalp. No globus, no anaesthesia. At my request she tries to get up, the effort succeeds by pushing her hands on the table in front of her, the patient stands for a moment on her legs, then falls back on the sofa.

While occupying the horizontal position, she can execute desired movements with her lower limbs. Deep and superficial reflexes are normal. She sleeps badly. She gets to sleep late at night and sleeps

---

[64] * Pain in the spine.

lightly; the patient wakes at the least noise and always spontaneously as soon as daylight comes.

The inability to walk has never lasted as long as this time.

The patient has been submitted to various treatments: medicines, massage, hydrotherapy and electricity, alone and in combination over a long period of time to no effect.

On the following 14 April, the patient was admitted to my clinic and I began treatment by suggestion on the same day.

I obtained and have only ever been able to obtain with her a very light hypnosis, a small degree of relaxation. However the patient proved to be sufficiently suggestible. Under the influence of my suggestions repeated on a daily basis her insomnia and aversion to food soon disappeared. From the 3rd day I introduced systematic exercises, first passive and then active, during the hypnotic state and after her sleep.

The effect obtained was fabulous. In fact from the 26 April, the patient was able to go from third floor of the apartment block she occupied down to the ground floor. This involved descending 52 stairs without holding on to the bannister.

On the 12 June she left my house much improved. She was able to take an hour's walk without any notable tiredness, was free of headaches and back pain, ate with appetite, could read for half an hour and occupy herself with some handwork without cerebral fatigue. Only the sweaty hands persisted. I recommended the patient to follow the regime of exercises in her own home and let me know how she was getting on from time to time.

My patient hasn't had a relapse of her motor asthenia. From time to time she has complained of a headache. The latest news dates from January 1894 and is good.

## OBS. 37.

MIXED FORM OF TWO GRAND NEUROSES: HYSTERIA AND NEURASTHENIA. NOTABLE PERSISTENT IMPROVEMENT.

On 14 June 1888 a colleague asked me to care for his niece, a young woman aged 23, who for some years had become a recluse in the paternal home and dared not go out.

She is an only child and has enjoyed excellent health since her earliest days. Her illness began at the age of twelve. Following a fright she was overtaken by a painful sensation in the region of her stomach, followed by noisy eructations. Since then the phenomenon has repeated itself in the form of fits accompanied by precordial anxiety.

These fits occur unexpectedly, in the event of any emotion, the very thought: "a fit is going to happen" suffices to bring it on.

The unwelcome noise of the eructation is very painful for the patient. At first it made her shun society and soon condemned her to remain in the house. The parents are very nervy, the father is choleric, however neither of them has suffered from serious nervous problems. No members of the family suffer from nerves.

*Present state,* 14 June 1888.

Young blond girl of medium height, pale, malnourished, lets me know that she is afraid to leave the house because she fears being surprised at any moment by noisy eructations. She complains of various symptoms which sometimes occur alone, sometimes in combination or alternately: vertigo, ringing in the ears, headaches, rachialgia, precordial anxiety, feeling as if she is going to vomit, lump in the throat which prevents her from eating certain food such as vegetables and meat (with the exception of beef steak) and heart palpitations.

She feels a painful point in her right breast, she even believes there might be a small tumour there and fears that it could be an indication of cancer. Sometimes spontaneously or following a sensation of precordial anxiety, her respiration accelerates and becomes difficult. These experiences have given her the idea that she will get asthma, an illness which caused the death of a paternal uncle. Her appetite is nil. The patient eats very little. Chronic constipation. Bowels only open in response to a douche. The effort necessary in excretion often gives rise to a feeling of general malaise and heart pain. Menstrual periods are regular, preceded by a state of sadness, dejection and bursts of tears. The patient goes to bed late. Her dreams make her frightened of sleeping, she often has nightmares. Her bedroom communicates with that of her parents. The door stays open and if she wakes during the night in a state of fear, she plucks up her courage by ceaselessly repeating "good night" to her parents. If they are slow in responding, she begins to scream in a loud voice, prompted by fear. She wakes up late in the morning feeling tired and with a heavy head. During the day, she occupies herself, sometimes feverishly for hours on end, with hobbies or sorting out her laundry. Sometimes in a sad or mournful dejected mood she does nothing at all, or gets agitated and tormented by anxiety, or again she gets carried away by a triviality. She has an irrational fear of storms, of all illnesses that she reads about or hears spoken of, and of darkness.

The family doctor who is also her uncle and other doctors and specialists after him, have examined her many times and have been of the unanimous opinion that she has no organic lesions. She has never wished to take drugs. She has always outrightly refused to take any medication. If I am only suffering from nerves, she argues, medicine can do nothing for me, only magnetism would be able to cure me. The parents, following the advice of the doctor, have never agreed until now to a treatment by magnetism. However since a psycho-therapy clinic was founded in Amsterdam, they finally ceded to the patient's wishes and allowed her to be treated by suggestion.

On examination which I carried out, I only noted functional nervous troubles of a hysterical and neurasthenic kind.

I told the patient that I could assure her of a cure if she consented to become an in-patient in my clinic for a while where I would treat her with hypnotism. At first she raised a few objections but gave way to my insistence that I would not treat her at home.

She made the journey from her home to the clinic by carriage in the evening. Her mother kept her company and shared her bedroom during the night.

The treatment began on 1st July 1888. I obtained, and was only able to obtain during the course of the treatment, a light hypnosis. However suggestibility in other circumstances was sufficient to gradually produce a marked improvement in her mental condition.

The bouts of eructations diminished in number and intensity, sleep and nutrition improved, various forms of anxiety began to disappear; however it wasn't before the 28 Dec. of that same year that I was able to get the patient to go out.

The first walk lasted a quarter of an hour. The patient was agitated, took large steps and was relieved to set foot in the clinic on her return.

From then on she walked every day if the weather wasn't too bad. However, it took months before she enjoyed her walks and before she dared to risk taking a walk alone on the roads in the middle of the day. The risk of an eructation would always occur and keep running through her mind.

On the 1st August 1889 she was sufficiently recovered to leave the clinic. However she still dared not return home because in her opinion the paternal house was too far from the clinic (a half hour's walk), and she feared she couldn't last out that long. Anxiety in her daily walk to or from the clinic might take hold of her or she might be surprised by an eructation. A flat was rented in the neighbourhood from where she gradually increased the length of her daily walks.

Finally on the 1st Dec. 1889 my patient definitively returned home.

During the course of the following year, I spread out the sessions more and more. The daily walks were continued.

Whereas the various symptoms described disappeared one after the other, others made their appearance such as: fear of getting into a carriage, of getting into a tram and of travelling on the railway, but they responded to appropriate suggestions.

In May 1891 my patient became engaged, then went to spend several months in the country where she continued to gain in strength and energy. She got married in Oct. 1892 and gave birth on 19 Sept. 1893 to a beautiful child.

During the last two years I have only seen the patient at very great intervals, everything is going well. On the last visit I made to the young mother, she was able to assure me of her excellent health, however she continued to have a holy horror of medicines.

## OBS. 38.

HYSTERO-NEURASTHENIA. MARKED IMPROVEMENT OBTAINED BY PSYCHOTHERAPY.

An unmarried lady aged 25 years, daughter of a very nervous mother and a choleric father had experienced much unhappiness in her childhood. Her parents didn't get on. She feared her father and adored her mother, who suffered a lot seeing her daughter ignored and neglected by her husband. The patient is of a sensitive nature, easily moved from a tender age. She hasn't had any serious illnesses, learned with ease, profited a great deal from her primary and secondary education and was destined by her father (a dental surgeon), against her will, to succeed him in his specialty. Miss Z. learned to overcome her aversion in order to please her mother and passed her examinations after assiduous and difficult studies.

She lost her parents one shortly after the other. Her mother's death, above all, troubled her greatly. A little after this event she was disturbed nervous of the hysterical and melancholic variety. However her condition gradually improved, she established herself as a dentist at the age of 20 years and succeeded in creating an excellent clientele.

On the 28 June 1892 she took a very hot foot-bath. Her companion told her that it was dangerous, in fact very dangerous to take a foot-bath during menstruation. She said she recalled a case where a bath taken under those conditions was followed by a death. Miss Z., who had her period just then, at first seemed unbothered by these words. However not long after going to bed, the remark which she had at first laughed off, began to have an unfortunate effect. She felt anxious, her heart started palpitating, then a feeling of tension in her neck was added followed by a dreadful anxiety, a relentless fear of dying or going mad. She didn't sleep the whole night long.

The doctor whom she consulted diagnosed acute cerebral anaemia and prescribed a fortifying diet and absolute rest. Her condition remained the same, it was treated — but in vain — the insomnia was resistant to strong doses of chloral which failed to help her, the doctor ended up by referring the patient to a hydrotherapy station in the province.

Far from curing the patient the hydrotherapy procedures irritated her. After a stay of four weeks, she returned to Amsterdam and asked her doctor to allow her to consult me.

12 Sept. 1892. *Present state.*

A small person looking frail, quite debilitated, pale mucosas. Is very agitated. She dares not go out alone as she is afraid of water. If her route is along a canal, she walks along the houses not daring to look at the water and at the same time feeling drawn towards it. She has to make an effort not to throw herself in. She is tormented by nosophobia, she is afraid of hearing about patients and illnesses and fears going mad. She dares not sleep alone. She often spends entire nights without shutting an eye. It's really rare for her to sleep well, she often has nightmares and an oppressive sensation in her chest. She knows she is asleep but she cannot wake herself up. Sometimes her sister, who shares her bedroom, sees that her sleep is disturbed and so she wakes her. If she isn't woken, the anxiety always increases, in the end she begins to scream and thus wakes herself up. Then she doesn't want to go back to sleep, she often fears going to sleep.

Already for a long time it has been impossible for her to eat, she has a pronounced disgust for food. Cloakroom-use retarded, constipation has been chronic since her infancy, she always feels embarrassed to absent herself from company as a result of prudery and timidity. Periods are regular but painful, if she isn't careful to take a purgative at those times, they slow down and only show after an adequate alvine[65] evacuation.

Bouts of precordial anxiety accompanied by heart palpitations and a sensation of tightness in the occipital region are very frequent. She often suffers from headaches. No globus or anaesthesias. No organic lesions.

I succeeded in calming the patient's anxiety, indicating to her that she simply suffers from a functional disorder and promising her a certain cure. Her hereditary neuropathic predisposition added to the intellectual overwork caused by the serious study required for her examinations and the successive loss of her father and mother, had succeeded in profoundly shaking her nervous equilibrium. Also her lady companion's remarks had given rise to a blossoming of nervous phenomena having alighted on a suitably prepared terrain.

I prescribed a diet and advised the patient to resume her consultations as soon as possible. I insisted that she come to see me every day, absolutely abstain from talking about her illness or her symptoms to whomever and that she confide her sorrows to me alone. A trial of hypnosis failed and raised her anxiety. So from that time onwards I didn't insist on inducing sleep. I contented myself

---

[65] • Intestinal.

with making my suggestions while she was awake, to raise her morale, and to regulate her life. Today (January 1894) Miss Z. is still continuing her treatment and although by all accounts much better, frankly, she isn't yet cured. The suggestive sessions that I initially gave her on a daily basis are no longer given more than 2 or 3 times a week and take up scarcely more than a quarter of an hour in the mornings.

So she is free of all her worries and leaves me every time feeling comforted and encouraged. From the third day of my treatment she continued her professional consultations and hasn't missed a day since then. Apart from some rare exceptions she sleeps well every night, alone and without a light, she no longer has nightmares or palpitations.

The fear of water is tenacious. However she no longer avoids the roads along the canal as she used to do, still the sight of water gives her a disagreeable feeling. She lets herself go to the theatre and concerts, she can read and hear about emotional things without it creating anxiety.

Her appetite continues to be capricious. She generally eats enough. Bowels open every two or three days.

## OBS. 39.

CONSTIPATION GVING RISE TO NERVOUS ATTACKS OF A NEURASTHENIC NATURE, IN A HEREDITARY PREDISPOSITION. MIXED TREATMENT BY MEDICINES AND SUGGESTION. CURE.

A retired civil servant underwent a radical operation on external haemorrhoids two months ago. The operation succeeded perfectly, however incessant painful tenesmus[66] had given rise to a state of agitation such that the patient himself demanded his admission to my clinic.

*Past history.*

A man nervous since birth, who had worked very hard and secured an honourable position as a result of his labour and conscientiousness. For some years, worries and family unhappiness have caused the reactivation of latent neurasthenic symptoms. Early retirement has been the consequence.

Hypochondriacal preoccupations have always tormented our patient, sometimes atonic gastro-intestinal phenomena suggest a stomach disease, sometimes episodes of palpitations and tachycardia simulate heart disease. Bouts of migraine, vertigo, rachialgia, have made him fear having brain involvement or possibly being subject to myelitis. In recent times he believed himself to be suffering from enteritis. He was experiencing alternate bouts of diarrhoea and constipation and a sensation of heaviness in the lower abdomen with tenesmus. And when an examination carried out by a colleague indicated haemorrhoids, the patient wasn't slow to demand a radical operation from his doctor.

The extirpation using thermo-cautery was very painful, however after three weeks the wound healed and the doctor reduced the frequency of his visits. It was then that the nervous phenomena

---

[66] * Continual or recurrent inclination to evacuate the bowels.

recurred, the painful tenesmus that had initially disappeared, reappeared. In answer to his complaints from which he didn't spare his doctor, that gentleman one day replied, that the pains only existed in his imagination. He lost all confidence in him. He had been prescribed a bromide potion to calm his nerves, some laudanum to kill the pain, and packets of powdered opium to combat insomnia.

*Present state.*

After a journey of two hours by rail, the patient arrived at my house at 7 o'clock in the evening on 11 August 1891. A 53-year-old man who seemed like a 65-year-old at least. Dull eyes, sweat dripping from his forehead, tired, exhausted and breathless, he insisted on lying down immediately. The journey had been very difficult for him, above all having to remain seated and hold back his tenesmus. He hadn't slept the whole of the previous night.

After the patient undressed and lay down I proceeded to examine him. The abdomen was distended, abdominal wall slightly soft, slightly depressible, painful to palpation beginning in the right hypochondrium at the top of the caecum and going all the way along the ascending and transverse colon.

The cutaneous tegument surrounding the anal orifice had a shiny red appearance and was scattered with small fissures. Every 2 or 3 minutes the tenesmus coming from the intestine caused the discharge of small quantities of faecal matter.

Urination infrequent and with difficulty. Pulse 110, weak. T. 37.8°C. The patient claimed his pulse was always about 100.

Appetite left nothing to be desired, except during the last few days. He ate a lot, mainly farinaceous food.

He had been forbidden vegetables, fruit, anything likely to produce a bowel movement.

The patient himself feared intestinal opening due to the tenesmus triggered by it and the fear that it would slow the healing of his wound.

Introducing my index finger into the anus, I noted that the overextended intestine appeared to be stuffed with hard friable faecal matter.

The patient is anxious. He is frightened of dying. He feels he is very ill, weak in the extreme. He is irritable to the highest degree, sleeps little and badly.

When I told him that before doing anything else it would be necessary to empty the intestine of its contents, he protested. He didn't want to believe that he was constipated, since a small quantity of faecal material emerged very time he experienced the tenesmus.

He demanded to be treated by hypnotism. I was able to calm him and give him a few hours sleep. The next day he felt a bit better, ate with appetite, however the tenesmus continued to torment him. It was only on the day after that I was able to get him to accept a warm water douche. A first evacuation of abundant, fetid, faecal material did him good and convinced him of the rightness of my advice. I followed the enema with a good dose of castor-oil which produced a fabulous outpouring on the following day.

The patient continued to feel relieved and much better than before. The tenesmus continued to occur all the time although to a lesser extent and the patient predicted that the phenomenon wouldn't be slow in returning. So I had recourse to hypnotic suggestion and I succeeded in procuring two hours light sleep for the patient every day. My repeated daily suggestions, lasting for a fortnight were completely realised. His cantankerous mood dissipated, he began to sleep better at night, moved his bowels regularly each day. The tenesmus was suppressed and he enjoyed a calm which was immediately apparent. His state of weakness and fatigue had given way to a feeling of well-being. He was able to remain sitting without pain, to walk without getting tired. On the 2nd day of treatment I declared him cured and he left my establishment happy but not satisfied. He specifically demanded to be put into a deep hypnotic state. He believed he would be cured by suggestion given in a deep sleep and his suggested sleep had scarcely passed the stage of light somnolence.

News that the patient provided me with a fortnight after he left confirmed his cure.

**OBS. 40.**

NEURASTHENIC HYPOCHONDRIA, CURE.

A young man aged 24, looking vigorous, robust and appearing to enjoy perfect health comes to consult me for sexual impotence. A single man, he lives with his mother who is a widow.

As a child he was always very nervous, irritable, easily carried away but never had any serious illness. He confesses to having been addicted to masturbation for a long time, a fact about which he is very worried. He left school early in order to learn the diamond cutting trade, a profession in which he soon excelled and which quickly procured an easy life for him. A love affair with his mother's maid made him a father at the age of 18. The fear that his mother would discover his lover's pregnancy extinguished his flame and was the cause of his first nervous problems which presented at that time.

Precordial anxiety, heart palpitations, nosophobia (fear of pulmonary phthisis, heart disease, tabes dorsals, blindness) caused him much suffering and made him consult various doctors and follow all sorts of treatments over a period of six years.

Various different drugs, electricity and hypnotism also took their turn in bearing the brunt of his treatment, which he tried without benefit.

Although the patient counted many nervous individuals in his family, neither of his parents had a serious nervous illness.

*Present state* 28 May 1892.

The patient is impressionable and easily moved. He has a lively imagination and quickly applies to himself all the signs and symptoms of illnesses he hears spoken of. At the moment he is preoccupied with the idea that he has an eye disease and is threatened with going blind. However a thorough examination carried out by a specialist revealed nothing abnormal, nothing more than a minor anomaly of refraction corrected by appropriate spectacles. The work of diamond cutting demands prolonged, tiring exercise of the eyes. If during his work the thought "I can't see anymore" comes to him, his eyes immediately close and he ceases to see. This phenomenon worries and obsesses him. He suffers a lot from heart palpitations and has been examined several times by different doctors who have all assured him that he has nothing to fear on that score. However he continues to doubt and is not at all reassured.

He was treated for a long time for gonorrhoea and was cured. An itching sensation at the orifice of the urethra occurs after urination and worries him a lot. Urine is clear, no chronic urethritis. Another thing which worried him was the lack of any voluptuous feeling during his first attempt at coitus following his cure. The *nisus coëundi*[67] gradually diminished from that time, above all after he noticed that coitus was followed by pains in his left hip. It was then that he first thought he was impotent. He maintains a relationship with a girl but hasn't been to see her for some time.

He is easily moved to anger, complains of having a bad memory, often has bouts of melancholy during which he would like to put an end to his life. He carries out his work automatically, but it is satisfactory. However the state of his eyes worries him, he fears that he will become infirm and incapable of work,

No hysterical stigmata. Good appetite, bowels open regularly. Sleep, sometimes excellent, sometimes doesn't happen at all.

---

[67] * Desire to have sex.

I explained to the patient that he was neurasthenic, that his case although serious was perfectly curable, and I prevailed upon him to take courage. I began treatment by hypnotic suggestion on the same day. The effect of my suggestions was very favourable.

After a few weeks there were no longer any symptoms other than a light asthenopia. From then on I continued to see him at greater intervals and at present (January 1894) his health leaves nothing to be desired. He is always cheerful and in good spirits although he has been out of work these last few months. This state of affairs has forced him to make a living from music which he practices as an amateur. Thanks to my care he has become a calm man, who knows how to deal with himself, and who has learnt auto-suggestion so that any nervous phenomena, whatever they may be, disappear quickly in response to his telling them to stop.

The hypnotic sleep obtained never got further than a light sleep.

## OBS. 41.

OBSESSIVE IDEA. CURE BY PSYCHO-THERAPY.

A worker, diamond cutter, unmarried and aged 25 years, son of nervous parents and counts many nervous people, mainly on the female side of his family.

He claims never to have been sick before the month of June 1888. He left school at the age of 17 and went into the profession of diamond cutting. He worked hard, never did anything excessive but permitted himself some fun from time to time.

In June 1888 he received a visit from a friend who had been suffering for some time from a cancerous? tumour on the left side of his neck and he showed it to him. It made a great impression. From that moment on, and at all hours, he mentally visualised the malignant tumour and he felt pain in the corresponding part of his own neck and couldn't stop himself from constantly touching it with his hand. He lost his cheerful disposition, became more and more morose, he avoided all society, no longer dared to read the gazette for fear of finding an article or allusion to the terrible affliction which obsessed him. Even while working the thought that he had cancer of the neck pursued him. He began to lose sleep and developed the habit of drinking a cognac in the evening in order to get to sleep. It was only in Nov. 1889 that he resolved to tell his doctor, who tried hypnotic suggestion over a period of six weeks, without being able to put the patient to sleep nor produce the slightest benefit.

On the 19 January 1890 the patient came to me and asked me to try to rid him of his idée fixe during hypnotic sleep.

After having put two or three other patients to sleep in his presence, by simple occlusion of their eyelids, I invited the patient to sit in an armchair that I placed in front of him. Scarcely was he seated then I gently closed his eyes and told him that he was already asleep, a suggestion which was perfectly realised within two minutes.

Suggestive catalepsy. Invited to open his eyes he made fruitless efforts, he wasn't able to do so.

From that first session the patient began to improve. The obsessional idea disappeared sometimes even for a period of several hours. From the third session he recovered his sleep at night. From then on I arranged for him to see me not more than once a week. At the end of the first month he lost the habit of bringing his hand to his neck all the time in order to check whether he had a tumour, he no longer felt pain in that part of his body. He began to go out again, to visit a cafe or theatre. However he still avoided reading his gazette, fearing the impression that any news touching on the subject of cancer might make.

During work, which was purely automatic, not requiring any mental effort, the obsessional idea still often insinuated itself into his brain.

I advised him to learn a foreign language during his leisure time and to mentally go over his lessons or repeat them out loud while he was at work, which would drive out the obsessional idea. He put my advice into practice and thus completely succeeded in getting rid of the idea. After a few months he was cured. During the summer of 1890 he went away for 4 weeks holiday and when he saw me on his return, he confirmed the persistence of his cure. I reviewed the patient in august 1894, he was in remarkably good health and completely free of the obsessional idea.

## OBS. 42.

INSOMNIA ACCOMPANIED BY FEAR OF GOING MAD IN A NEURASTHENIC; MARKED IMPROVEMENT.

A single artist, aged 41 years, a painter-decorator, had been obsessed for some weeks with the fear of going mad.

He had been sleeping very little or not at all for a long time. He went to bed late, got up early, wasn't exactly what one would call sober; however he wasn't a heavy drinker and worked from morning till night.

He lost his parents at a very young age. He doesn't remember ever having had a serious illness. After receiving his primary education he became an apprentice in a painter-decorator's studio in a large theatre. He was ambitious in his work and had the good fortune to succeed his master. To get to that position he had had to do the impossible, he worked himself into the ground for years on end, only allowed himself a few hours sleep at night, never took any rest or holidays, in short a time arrived when he became neurasthenic due to overwork. He lived in a state of continual agitation, everything had to be done quickly. He often didn't sleep the whole night long, sometimes for just one or two hours.

On getting up he is more tired than when he went to bed. During the course of the day his fatigue diminishes, he feels best in the evenings. Above all his eyes are painful and tired. His appetite is normal, bowels move regularly.

Treatment by hypnotic suggestion from 13 July to 30 august 1891. The patient became somnolent and spent two hours every day in that state which did him an enormous amount of good. Above everything else he appreciated the calm which hypnosis procured for him. Under this regime his sleep at night improved, he slept regularly 4 to 6 hours. The fear of going mad disappeared completely. He was unable to continue treatment due to his occupation, but he promised himself to come back if ever the insomnia returned.

## OBS. 43.

RESISTANT INSOMNIA, AGORAPHOBIA, THOUGHTS OF SUICIDE. MARKED IMPROVEMENT THROUGH SUGGESTION.

A married lady aged 36 years, counting several members of her family affected by severe neurasthenia and hysteria, having suffered for some years from agrypnia[68] and agoraphobia. In recent times she has been haunted by the fear of committing suicide. Her doctor prescribed a special diet, mainly in view of her gastric symptoms which were not very serious, and treated the insomnia with narcotics. She takes 1 or 2 grammes of sulfonal every night.

As I had treated her sister by hypnotic suggestion (grand hysteric) with great success, she asked to come under my care on 20 Sept. 1892.

---

[68].Syndrome characterized by loss of sleep and permanent motor and autonomic hyperactivation.

Very agitated she confessed that she was frightened of sleeping as profoundly as her sister, she dared not look me in the eye, absolutely didn't want to be put to sleep, she feared that I wouldn't be able to wake her up. I tried to calm her agitation as much as possible and I reassured her concerning her sleep. I promised not to put her to sleep, that she would only feel a state of calm, light torpor, that she would be able to open her eyes spontaneously whenever she liked.

On that I asked her to close her eyes. Her eyelids batted for a few moments and then closed. I gave her the suggestion of sleeping at night without recourse to narcotics, of having the courage to go out alone, of even on that day returning home unaccompanied and finally no longer having gastric symptoms.

Waking up after ten minutes, she assured me that she'd heard everything I said word for word, but that she had tried to reply in vain, her tongue refused to work. She had felt relaxed and agreeable calm, her agitation had disappeared. The next day at my request, she handed over her supply of sulfonal.

The patient put all my suggestions perfectly into practice, to the extent that she felt cured after a few days. Everything went wonderfully until on the 15 Oct. she was frightened by an encounter with a woman in my waiting room who was in the midst of a nervous crisis. Although calmed by appropriate suggestions that I gave her some moments later, the incident was followed by a sleepless night. A 2nd and 3rd night passed in the same manner without sleep and were followed by the reawakening of her anxieties, and the patient insisted forcefully that I allow her to resume her narcotics. I agreed to give permission and advised her to take 1 gramme of sulfonal on going to bed; if she woke during the night she would be free to take another gramme. I added that I was relying entirely on her good faith and that I was sure she would only have recourse to sulfonal as a last resort.

19 Oct. The patient feels altogether reassured. She slept well after only one dose of medicine and feels herself entirely rid of her fears.

20 Oct. Good night. No need for sulfonal. No fear of open spaces.

Since then I've only seen the patient infrequently. She keeps her sulfonal in reserve and doesn't use it.

January 1894. The patient continues to be free of insomnia, to eat healthily, to enjoy good digestion, she no longer has symptoms of agoraphobia . On the other hand she has had incidental symptoms of nosophobia, fear of cancer, of hydrophobia and other diseases, from time to time. Luckily her auto-suggestibility is diminished and easily vanquished by her suggestibility to others. Her husband under my instruction possesses a sufficient degree of influence over his wife to clam her when the need arises and to guide her.

## OBS. 44.

FEAR OF OPEN SPACES, HORROR OF HEIGHTS, NOSOPHOBIA IMPROVED BY PSYCHO-THERAPY.

One of my colleagues, an army doctor, asked me if I would kindly look after his brother, a young man of 22 years, suffering from fear of open spaces. The phenomenon began at the age of 15 years when he saw a mason on the point of slipping from a scaffold on a high building who just managed to save himself from a mortal fall. From that time a feeling of anxiety took hold of him whenever he wanted to cross a public square or cross a bridge or even walk along a wide unpopulated road. He can't look up towards the roof of a church or tall building without getting vertigo and running the risk of falling.

He has had to give up his studies as an architect and has become an apprentice in a bookshop.

In his family history I learned that his mother is a chronic arthritic and his father is a very nervous man. The patient is an orderly young man who has never engaged in any debauchery, he hasn't had any serious illness besides a keratitis followed by a central spot which bothers him a great deal, especially during prolonged reading, when he gets a sense of heaviness in his forehead. He has a moderate myopia corrected with appropriate glasses. He has suffered with constipation for a long time. This problem has been cured by a special diet, massage and salt water enemas.

The patient understands perfectly that his fear is illusory, however it is stronger than he is.

*Present state* 6 Oct. 1891.

Accompanied by his sister, the young man looks perfectly healthy, but very agitated and shaken by heartbeats which I can hear from some distance, he comes to see me just as I am hypnotising another patient. The sight of this spectacle shocks him and he needs to support himself on the back of a nearby chair in order not to fall.

Examination reveals no organic lesion. Besides fear of spaces he complains of not being able to pay serious attention to any work because of all sorts of horrible thoughts that cross his mind. Any talk or reading alluding to illness but above all mental illness obsesses him for several days, his thoughts keep returning to and ruminating over what he has heard. If he passes by a charcuterie, he conjures up a whole scene of butchery and feels anxious, is frightened of blood, knives etc.

A first session which I gave on the same day visibly calmed him and from the third day he was already able to leave unaccompanied, but armed with a stick.

After a fortnight a very notable improvement had been achieved, his self-confidence gradually grew, his sensitivity to things people talked about which previously completely upset him was reduced and the patient was able to resume the work he had abandoned for several months. From then on I spaced out the sessions but I continued regular treatment until the June 1892. The hypnotic state never surpassed the stage of somnolence.

In autumn 1892 he felt sufficiently well to seriously contemplate opening a bookshop, an idea which he put into practice in May 1893, he described his condition to me in these terms:

"I can now work all day without getting tired and without any preoccupations. I walk regularly at least two hours per day without having to avoid wide empty roads, and also without avoiding large squares. I have to confess that sometimes a little anxiety rears its head but I always succeed perfectly in conquering my enemy, without quickening my pace. I think of you, I call myself a coward and I continue on my way without diverting. Walking in broad daylight is always less trying than walking in the evening. I have great confidence in my future, I am much better at managing myself and if I am still not completely free of anxiety, I can assure you that I feel so well that if my previous state had been what it is now, of course I would never have thought of consulting a doctor."

**OBS. 45.**

NERVOUS SYMPTOMS, OBSESSIONAL IDEAS TRIGGERED BY PREGNANCY IN A HEREDITARY PREDISPOSITION. CURE BY HYPNOTIC SUGGESTION.

Mrs N., married for several moths, complains of insomnia and various types of phobia. She is 22 years old, seems very fit, loves her husband very much and believes she is 12 to 16 weeks pregnant.

*Family history.*

The father died young. The mother is a hysteric. One sister was under my care and cured of obsessional ideas. A brother is alcoholic. A maternal aunt is insane, another aunt is a hysteric.

*Personal history.*

No serious childhood illnesses. Mrs N. was always a nervous child. As a young girl she was timid. She spent a year in boarding school in a town in Germany. During the first weeks of her stay in that school she was unhappy, refused to eat, and they were on the point of sending her home due to homesickness. However a turnaround occurred, she regained her good spirits and her appetite and fitted in completely with her new environment. At the end of the year she returned to Holland with regrets. She never had nervous problems before her marriage.

*Present state* 15 sept. 1892.

Menstrual periods always regular haven't occurred since the end of May. From that time, she feels as if she changed, she lives in a state of continual agitation, moments of overexcitement alternate with periods of depression.

She is disgusted by her usual occupations, she neglects her housework, no longer enjoys reading, handwork, shuns society.

About four weeks ago, her husband — a naval officer — misunderstanding her condition and wishing to tease her, drew his sabre and made as if to strike her. This badinage far from having the desired effect, notably to distract and amuse her, put her into a mad fear. Since then she has been obsessed by the fear of weapons, sharp instruments, scissors, pins. At the same time she feels attracted to touch these objects and worries that she will use one to kill herself. She also insists that they be carefully hidden away to keep them from herself. She is nosophobic, cannot hear of illnesses or accidents without becoming full of anxiety. She eats and sleeps badly. Heart palpitations. Occasional headaches.

On examination I note probable pregnancy and the absence of organic lesions.

I received the patient in my house on the 24 September following and I treated her by hypnotic suggestion until early December. From the beginning of the treatment her sleep and nutrition normalised. The obsessional ideas gradually disappeared and side by side with this improvement in her general condition the patient resumed various occupations, handwork, reading, taking part in board-games. From the month of November she took a good walk every day, accompanied my wife and myself to the theatre or a concert from time to time. She didn't stop her sessions, notwithstanding the advanced state of her pregnancy and a five hour railway journey (here and back). She gave birth happily on the 22 February to a beautiful child whom she had the painful misfortune to lose fifteen day later.

The latest news that I received from my interesting patient dates from the 27 April following. She continues to keep well, sleeps perfectly and remains free of her fears.

## OBS. 46.

OBSESSIVE IDEA SUPPRESSED BY HYPNOTIC SUGGESTION.

A clerk of the court of first instance in a provincial town, single man aged 39 years has had two attacks of gout. The arthritic diathesis is hereditary in his family as is the nervous one.

Ten years ago during a court session he was suddenly struck by a sensation of precordial anxiety, a lump in his throat made it absolutely impossible for him to read out the judicial acts which he was charged to do. Since then nothing similar has happened.

Now in a few days time the court will have to pass judgement on an affair which has attracted much publicity. A distinguished audience will be in court and a famous advocate from the capital will be in charge of the case for the defence.

Our clerk feels uncomfortable and is obsessed by the idea that he will not have the necessary aplomb, won't be able to do his duty, in short that the same scene as in the past will repeat itself..

He asks me to give him a suggestion which will put him in a state where he will be able to fulfil the necessary functions.

The famous session will take place in five days time.

I do my best to get the patient right and I succeed perfectly in immediately putting him to sleep. After a half hour of sleep during which I assure him that he will be perfectly calm and in control of himself in the forthcoming session, his anxiety is very much allayed. The next day and the day before the session I repeat the hypnotic suggestion. Several days later I had the satisfaction of learning that my suggestions had an excellent effect, notably that the session had taken place without any undue incident.

## OBS. 47.

NERVOUS TREMOR, OBSESSIONAL IDEA. CURE BY HYPNOTIC SUGGESTION.

A law student aged 26 years, from a family of neuropaths but without any serious personal history, had overworked mainly during the two previous years in order to prepare for his examinations. His health has always been good, he sleeps well at night, doesn't indulge in any excesses. However he has been worried for some time by a tremor in his hands which happens when he extends them or even when he thinks about doing so. Far from diminishing, the worry has gradually increased to the point of obsession.

Observing him while he speaks to me, I see the trembling start up. When I ask him to extend both his hands, he executes the movement which is followed by a very marked tremor, ceasing the moment that he lets his arms fall back.

I gave four sessions of hypnotic suggestion to the patient at weekly intervals. It seemed to me that the first session hadn't achieved the smallest influence over the subject, or at least he didn't seem to be asleep. I contented myself with making the suggestion: "You will no longer be preoccupied with this trembling, it's nothing, it'll pass!" However I noted improvement the following week. In a second session I obtained the charmed state, in a third deep sleep. From the fourth session the trembling was no more and didn't recur in the following five months

A few days before taking his doctoral theses, the patient presented with a relapse. I resumed the treatment and after several days everything was back in order. He took his thesis, received his doctorate and all anxiety on the subject of his trembling disappeared.

## OBS. 48.

VARIOUS NEUROPATHIC TROUBLES: INSOMNIA, DEPRESSION, NOSOPHOBIA, IN A HEREDITARILY PREDISPOSED PERSON. CURE OF SYMPTOMS BY HYPNOTIC SUGGESTION.

A slim fair-haired girl, well built, of robust health but very nervous, aged 21 years, consulted me asking to be cured of her state of nerves. Miss B. had a serious family history of nervous problems.

She complained of having uncontrollable anxiety and of living in continual agitation from the moment that anything whatever interfered with her normal daily routine.

An invitation from friends to a concert given to her several days in advance would make her anxious, stop her from sleeping, make her burst into tears, notwithstanding the fact that she adores music and very much likes to mix socially. She doesn't understand herself, she is oversensitive. When she was still a little girl going to catechism, she sometimes had this same anxiety. For example the pastor's direction to never do wrong, a recommendation made to everyone, struck her particularly. She felt his words were targeted specifically at her and for days on end she would suffer from this imaginary accusation and become obsessed with it.

If she opened a door inadvertently, the idea took hold that someone in the room was going to get cold from the draught, would perhaps die, and that she would have been the cause of it all. She couldn't hear talk of any kind of illness or read about one, or hear of an accident happening to anybody, without feeling immediately that she was stricken by the same malady or feeling pain in the limb involved.

She has all sorts of fears, gets upset over nothing. Like Miss B. she lives in a provincial town some distance away. I suggested that she come and spend a few weeks in Amsterdam in order to follow a course of treatment.

After a few days she came to see me with her mother who asked me to provide the necessary care for her daughter.

On the same day I put the patient to sleep for the first time, she appeared very suggestible. The sessions were repeated on a daily basis and had a favourable effect on her mental state. In fact after a few days her sleep at night was absolutely normal. Her pathological fears gradually dissipated, the sad mood disappeared, the continuous agitation and morbid preoccupations were lost.

The patient takes part in conversation and isn't bothered by a thousand things that previously upset her. She occupies herself with housework, handcraft and reading, spends part of the day walking, makes visits, accompanies her mother or friends to shows and concerts without the least anticipatory anxiety.

After three weeks treatment I spaced out the sessions more and more and after six weeks I allowed the patient, now perfectly recovered, to return home.

I have had news of Miss B. from time to time. Eighteen months have already gone by since this cure without any sign of relapse.

## OBS. 49.

MELANCHOLIA, OBSESSIVE IDEAS, SUICIDAL AND HOMICIDAL IMPULSES. CURE OBTAINED BY THE SUGGESTIVE METHOD.

M.W. is an employee in a commercial business which he entered as an office boy. He is married, 46 years old and father of four children. Coming from a family of neuropaths he has suffered from nervous symptoms from a young age.

Addicted to onanism as a young boy, he managed to stop himself indulging in this perverse practice in good time. It was fear that cured him of it. Notably reading a pamphlet on the subject of masturbation and its consequences turned him away from his vice.

He has always been of a gloomy disposition, is not very expansive, married young, never indulged in any excesses and became an enthusiastic, reliable and exemplary office worker. He has served the same boss for nearly thirty years.

About three years ago M.W. began to have neurasthenic symptoms, such as headaches, excessive emotionality, timidity, anxieties, getting carried away by things and aboulia.

He continued with his work as best he could for some months, until in the end he could no longer do it,

The doctor who treated him prescribed bromides, the patient didn't show any improvement. He was on the point of quitting his job, leaving the town and withdrawing to the countryside when a friend got him to consult me.

*Present state* 7 August 1891.

A man of medium height, well built, with an anxious shifty-eyed look, very agitated, comes to me accompanied by his wife.

He complains, tearfully, of being ceaselessly haunted by the idea of committing suicide or going mad. He has a sensation of tightness in his head, a continuous constriction across his forehead and temples which starts when he wakes up in the morning and doesn't stop until about evening time. His work no longer interests him, everything irritates him. He only thinks of his own inner state. He eats regularly and well, he always feels a little less miserable after a good meal. He goes to bed early and sleeps deeply, has no dreams. He wakes at six o'clock in the morning and immediately feels assailed by his black ideas. They are terrible, these ideas, since they compel him to pounce on his wife and cut her throat. He has been able to keep them in check until now, but he fears that they will take hold of him more and more strongly and that one day he will do it.

However he loves and cherishes his wife who cares for him selflessly, and nothing bothers him so much as the knowledge that her death would leave his family bereft of everything.

He stays in bed ruminating over these dark ideas until eight o'clock, gets up, has breakfast and goes shopping in town in order to kill time and try to forget himself.

I undertook treatment by suggestion on the same day. I obtained a state of somnolence and used it to calm the poor man. I urged him to resume his bookkeeping work as soon as possible, to get up regularly in the morning at six o'clock and then to go for a one to 1½ hour walk before breakfast, after having washed in cold water. I repeated my suggestive sessions every day and continued them for more than five months. The patient's condition gradually improved, he went back to work from the third day of treatment. At first he worked robotically, so to speak, however without making errors in his calculations. Little by little his interest returned and a normal state was reestablished. Black ideas in the mornings continued to torment him for a long time. However from the month of February 1892 M.W. felt completely free of his compulsions and his melancholy. He felt altogether changed. On coming home from the office in the evening and after having had dinner he looked after his children, corrected their homework, played with them or even accompanied his wife to the theatre. On waking up in the mornings no more heaviness in his head, he felt rested and began his day with a better disposition.

The cure wasn't belied until the end of July 1893. During the heatwave in the summer, the melancholic condition recurred with the same symptoms as before. The patient came to see me immediately and I resumed the treatment.

From the first sessions M.W. felt a marked improvement, he was able to continue his work. However his sate of psychological depression was only completely vanquished in the early days of January 1894. Now (August 1894) he is perfectly well.

## OBS. 50.

NERVOUS DYSPEPSIA, REFRACTORY TO DIFFERENT DRUG TREATMENTS, CURED BY SUGGESTION IN A WAKING STATE.

A dealer aged 37 years, single, frail looking, pale and debilitated, extremely thin, came to ask my advice on his case diagnosed as chronic gastritis by several doctors whom he had consulted.

*Family history.*

He is the son of a healthy mother and neuropathic father who died in 1877. Three children in the family died at a young age. One son died at the age of 19 from a stomach condition (nervous?). A daughter is still living but is often sick and suffers a lot from stomach problems.

*Personal history.*

The onset of his illness dates from 1868. He was at boarding school, thirteen years old, and had the misfortune to fall on his nose. This accident was followed by vomiting. He remembers clearly that he didn't have a headache or pain in his nose. From that time on his stomach has always been the "locus minoris resistentiae"[69]. In 1877 and 1878 after the death of his father he suffered a great deal with his stomach. Since then, whether precipitated by emotions or overwork, or even under the influence of certain atmospheric changes, relapses of this condition have often occurred.

In the month of Sept. 1892, an emotional state gave rise to a relapse of his illness which he still suffers from at the present time.

The symptoms which appear following when he becomes emotional are first: a sense of tension above the eyes extending towards the temporal region and top of the head, which turns into a headache. Shortly afterwards stomach pain and precordial palpitations are added. If the stomach pain is less severe, it is accompanied by some acid reflux, if more severe nausea, then vomiting not preceded by nausea and followed by diarrhoea and constipation. These symptoms are followed by anorexia, he refuses to eat, gradually gets weaker and feels tired all the time. Then he has difficulty in reading, his eyes get tired and bother him if he persists in trying to read.

If atmospheric changes take place at the outbreak of the syndrome, the symptoms described are preceded by a coryza[70].

The patient has been under the care of several renowned doctors without gaining any serious or persistent benefit. He was advised

---

[69] * Place of least resistance.

[70] * A cold.

as a last resort to go abroad and look for less tiring work in the middle of Europe.

*Present state* 26 December 1892.

Last September, following an emotion, the patient had a relapse of his gastritis and had to stay in bed for several weeks. He resumed work just a few days ago. He is following a diet composed of dairy products for breakfast, then during the day two fresh raw eggs and two or three glasses of milk and finally a dish of beans and a small amount of cold fat-free meat for dinner. He doesn't smoke, drinks very little wine, an occasional glass of beer. He lives like a monk, leaving his flat for the office and returning home immediately after work. He is armed with a flannel belt around the region of his stomach. He rubs this region morning and evening with hot brandy. Medication: a dose of sel de Carlsbad in early morning, and some packets of bismuth subnitrate.

At the moment he has no pain, he is free of digestive troubles and his bowels move regularly every morning. He sleeps well at night. Also everything would be better if he wasn't living in a continual trance and if he wasn't threatened by a return of his symptoms at the least infraction of his diet which he dared to allow himself. The slightest deviation from his diet is revenged by tension above his eyes followed by coryza and the whole series of previously described symptoms.

One of his friends whom I cured of a nervous problem advised him to come to see me, so he asked me to examine him. He absolutely accepts that he is nervous, but he is convinced that he has a stomach disease.

A thorough examination instituted on the same day and continued on the following two days led to the conclusion that there were no organic lesions of the stomach.

On the 29 December 1892 I begin treatment by suggestion. The patient is refractory to the suggestion of sleep; however he feels during his session (of a quarter to half an hour) a sense of restfulness, of wellbeing. He succeeds in concentrating his attention on my suggestions and distancing himself from all other thoughts. After the first sessions the patient gave up his flannel belt and his brandy rubs and gradually introduced changes in his diet so that by the end of the first month he was eating normally, bread, butter, and boiled eggs for breakfast, bread and cold meat ( preferably bacon) for lunch, and a full dinner (composed of soup, vegetables, meat or fish and dessert) and a supper of bread and ham, in addition 1½ to 2 litres of milk per day. He abstained completely from wine, liqueurs and beer. He gave up all medication, went about his business regularly, undertook moderate exercise, a one hour walk mornings and evenings. All without feeling the least indisposition.

From the earliest days I only gave my suggestions once a week and from the month of April, I only saw my patient twice a month. He developed an embonpoint and felt that he couldn't be better. During the course of the year he underwent some strong emotions, he ran the risk of relapsing many times, he even allowed himself a fortnight's holiday in October 1893 during which he failed to follow my diet and let himself drink German beer and a good glass of vin de Rhin, all without feeling the least dyspeptic symptoms.

I see the well patient now at very long intervals.

## A. GROUP III.

### Mental illnesses.

In dealing with this group, it seemed interesting to review the opinions of other equally competent authors and conscientious observers, who's judgement was authoritative in these matters, namely Messrs Forel, Aug. Voisin and Bernheim.

The mentally ill — we cite Professor Forel[71] — " are the least suggestible of all men; the seriously mentally ill are not suggestible at all. This results simply from the fact that states of arrest or morbid irritation acquire such intensity in the brains of the mentally ill that they cannot be parted from them by suggestion. Even if one succeeds in hypnotising a mentally ill person, most of the therapeutic suggestions will not be realised or will only be realised for a short space of time. Above all those suggestions addressed to delusional ideas will be the least successful. A mentally ill woman, Mrs X. believed herself to be a certain Mrs Y. I succeeded in putting her to sleep and in suggesting sleep and a good appetite, and even giving her post-hypnotic hallucinations which she realised perfectly. However when I assured her

---

[71] Aug. forel. Der Hypnotismus etc. 2e Auflage 1891. S. 101 u. 106.

during hypnotic sleep, and very forcefully, that she knew perfectly well that she was Mrs. X. and not Mrs. Y., and that this conviction had been an absurd delusional idea, which she could only now laugh at; she shook her head negatively throughout the time I was talking to her, in order to show that she didn't accept that suggestion.

" The brain is an instrument which we make use of in suggestion. In the mentally ill, this instrument is spoiled, malfunctions, doesn't work. The setbacks experienced with mental illnesses are evidence that hypnotic force resides in the brain of the hypnotised person and not that of the hypnotiser. In short here is my opinion:

" It is undeniable that certain forms of mental trouble, not too serious or generalised, can be improved and even cured by suggestion, if the patient possesses a very suggestible brain and if the operator knows how to handle suggestion well. Wettersrand has even succeeded in curing several cases of epilepsy, some minor cases of melancholia and hypochondriasis, by suggestion.

De Jong from the Hague and Aug. Voisin from Paris report analogous successes. However I do not understand Voisin's violently applied hypnosis and the cases that he describes seem for the most part to concern hysteria. But I and my colleague Doctor Von Speyr of Bern and others, have obtained some very remarkable successes. The great difficulty resides in the patient's lack of attention, in his inaccessibility and in the intensity of the morbid irritations."

At the International Congress of Hypnotism held in Paris in 1889[72], Doctor Aug. Voisin was invited to give a report on: "The indications for hypnotism and hypnotic suggestion in the treatment of mental illnesses and allied states." He expressed himself in these terms:

"I said several years ago that it would be wonderful if all the mentally ill were hypnotisable. Experience that I have acquired since then confirms me in that opinion.

Indeed, nothing is more satisfying than to have the means of relieving a mentally ill person of his delusional ideas and hallucinations in a short period of time, sometimes two or three sessions. There's a task to be undertaken, in order to disarm the incredulity of doctors who have no faith in the art of healing.

The impossibility of hypnotising the mentally ill was, you are aware, considered to be an absolute, before my first trials in 1880 on those suffering from acute mania.

Since then, success having encouraged my efforts, I tried out hypnotism on all the mentally ill in my service and I am very happy to have been able to hypnotise a certain number,

---

[72] Comp. Comptes-Rendus du premier congrès etc. Paris. 1891. Octave Doin. P. 146 et suiv.

around 10%. I hope to reach a higher tally, by perfecting and extending the techniques which I use.

I have successively applied this treatment to all the associated states: mental illnesses, moral troubles, vices, lower leanings, theft, abuse of drink, abuse of drugs, onanism, defects of memory and intelligence either congenital or acquired, convulsive attacks, sensory troubles or sensation in general, neuralgias, contractions, and intellectual and psychological disturbances which occur during menstruation.

One mustn't pretend that great patience isn't required for this treatment and the investment of a large amount of time. I have had to remain at the side of of several patients for two or three hours before succeeding in putting them to sleep. The hypnotic procedures have to be varied and the sessions may need to be started again eighteen or twenty times before giving up on success.

The degree of hypnotic sleep required is lethargy or somnambulism, but lethargy is much preferable; suggestion however can transform somnambulism into lethargy.

Once the first sleep is obtained the patient should be allowed to sleep for half an hour to an hour. Suggestion, which is the corollary of hypnotism and the basis of this therapeutic method, should only be employed in the second session.

To begin with suggestions should be limited, thus they shouldn't concern a delusional idea or sensory hallucination. Only in later sessions should one undertake to try to influence these states of mind.

In my practice suggestions given simultaneously in too great a number give rise to a noticeable malaise which is reflected in stiffening of the facial muscles, and they are less well executed on awakening. Moreover the patient shouldn't be woken up immediately after the suggestion has been made. He should be left in peace for a quarter or half an hour so that he can take in the suggestion and, so to speak, let it penetrate.

Sometimes I let very agitated and hallucinated mentally ill patients sleep for 12 to 23 hours at a time or even several days.

The suggestions should be made in a loud voice, formulated in a precise way and articulated with conviction and authority. The patient must be told to no longer hear such and such a voice or noise, see strange things such as animals or shadows, be aware of such a smell or have such a delusional idea.

It must be insisted that all these ideas are false, that they result from their illness, that they will get better, that they are cured and finally that they will continue to be healthy.

One sometimes observes on the physiognomy of hypnotised mentally ill patients an obvious frown when one makes a particular suggestion which is contrary to their own ideas. One has to insist until the patient acquiesces by word or gesture which indicates that the suggestion has succeeded.

It also sometimes happens that the suggestion is efficacious although the hypnotised patient has indicated that he will not obey.

I think that it should be an absolute principle to never suggest to a hypnotised person, an illusion, a hallucination, or any bad idea or harmful action and to only give good advice: to obey, to work, to think of the good, to do good, to detest badness and vice, to be agreeable, to be useful, to love his family and those around him. One should guard against making the hypnotised person into an experimental subject and a curiosity.

In addition, it is essential to never say in front of the hypnotised person that his illness is serious or incurable, on the contrary one must clearly state that his pain isn't serious and will get better.

There is one more point to which I particularly call your attention, it is to never hypnotise patients and to never make suggestions in front of other patients.

It is indispensable for the hypnotised person to remain isolated during his sleep, so that he will not be open to suggestions in opposition to your own. This measure is particularly essential in a service for neuropaths and the mentally ill, where malicious and wicked ideas are so common.

Thus I noted that some of the other patients suggested to the hypnotised ones that that they should no longer allow me to put them to sleep "because they were being used as my puppets", and I had a great deal of difficulty in destroying that suggested idea.

Acting on the above principles I applied therapeutic suggestion to the treatment of the mentally ill and the nervous in my service and in my private practice.

One can achieve cure of visual, auditory, olfactory, taste, and general sensory hallucinations in these patients and remarkably various delusional ideas as well."

Let us now present Professor Bernheim's words as expressed in his excellent work: Hypnotism, Suggestion, Psychotherapy:[73]

---
[73] Etudes nouvelles. P. 223.

" At first sight it seems that suggestion which addresses itself to the mind should be able to cure mental illnesses easily. This is a mistake! A fixed idea is often more difficult to uproot than a painful sensation. Even though I have tried many times to cure melancholia, hypochondria, obsessional illness, mania, delusions of persecution, I have always failed.

During their acute phases the mentally ill are in general difficult if not impossible to hypnotise. It is true that some maniacs have been able to be calmed by a vigorous suggestion during their florid phases. But the disease itself and its evolution isn't influenced. So even if one manages to hypnotise mentally ill people in the intervals between crises, I do not believe that one can prevent a relapse. For example two years ago, I treated a young American girl suffering from intermittent attacks of lypemania[74] lasting about ten to fifteen days, with intervals of three weeks during which the her cheerfulness and remarkable intelligence returned. The illness is hereditary.

I was able to hypnotise the patient, she was very compliant with suggestion, full of hope and confidence, she believed herself cured. But the crisis reappeared, as usual, before the

---

[74] *Melancholia.

state of mind solicited by suggestion had been able to be conjured.

The truly mentally ill are not curable by suggestion, since what dominates in them is auto-suggestion. If they were suggestible, they wouldn't be mentally ill. The organ of thought must be sane for psycho-therapy to act effectively upon it. There is something in the brain of the mentally ill that we don't understand, something which fatally disturbs that modality, something against which all our means of action remain impotent."

The results obtained by us are mainly in agreement with the views expressed by Professor Forel. One could say in general that it is no easy task for psycho-therapy to achieve favourable results in the treatment of the mentally ill, and that it has to face many setbacks in order to achieve, here and there, some rare amazing success.

Equipped with the necessary medical tact, suggestion can be applied in a number of cases of mental illness without exposing the patient to an exacerbation of their condition. The improvement et casu quo[75] the cure, could not have been obtained other than with the help of a propitious milieu

---

[75] *And in this case.

and a psychological operator who had broken with hypnotic practices and was armed with exceptional patience.

Suggestive therapy is particularly indicated in the psychoneuroses, mental aberrations with no organic cause, functional psychoses, especially in patients who have insight into their illness. However, even in cases of mental illness resulting from anatomical lesions of the cerebro-spinal nervous system, suggestion can be a precious tool in the hands of the psychiatrist.

**OBS. 51.**

NERVOUS ATTACKS. NIGHT TERRORS IN A HEREDITARILY PREDISPOSED CHILD. VERY MARKED IMPROVEMENT.

Eve is 10 years old. She is small for her age, a brown haired girl with big eyes overlooked by long eyelashes, of a delicate complexion. Her father died of chest trouble, her mother is noticeably run down, a very nervous woman subject to hemicrania[76]. Not a week passes without her staying in bed for at least one day due to her headache. Psychoses and nervous illnesses affect several members of the family. Eve has an eight-year-old sister in excellent health, robust and appearing to be her elder. The two go to school together, they are in the same class. Whereas the younger follows her lessons perfectly and without difficulty, Eve

---

[76] * Chronic headache always occurring on the same side of the face and head.

only goes to class in order to have a bit of fun. She knows how to read and write, isn't strong on arithmetic. She knows how to knit, however knitting tires her out and irritates her. She stays as close to her mother as possible. In the afternoons, as soon as mummy has finished her housework and can allow herself a little rest, Eve places herself next to her, puts her head on her mother's knees and goes to sleep. This sleep does her an infinite amount of good. She sleeps badly at night and has done so for a long time. Last year during the summer she had a very serious fright and her nervous symptoms date from that time. She has a capricious appetite, sometimes gluttonous, sometimes anorexic. Nervous fits: grimacing face, biting action, clenched hands accompanied by loss of consciousness, occur from time to time. These fits are preceded by a particular sensation which she describes as a cloud rising up from her feet to her throat. Bouts of headaches happen nearly every day, the pains are localised above the eyes and at the top of her head. She gets frightened by the slightest thing. In the evenings at 7.30pm. she lies down next to her little sister with whom she shares a bed. Whereas her sister isn't slow in getting to sleep, Eve stays awake, most often feeling frightened without knowing why. Sometimes she imagines herself seeing black men who threaten her and want to harm her, so she begins to tremble and scream in a loud voice. She doesn't go to sleep before her mummy goes to bed around midnight, who sleeps in the adjoining bedroom. Sleep is never calm, always troubled with dreams. On waking the child is often soaked in sweat.

The family doctor and a specialist in children's illnesses have treated her without achieving any change in her condition. On the 4 Oct. 1892 the mother confided her child to my care.

Like most children Eve seems very suggestible. I don't put her to sleep. I simply ask her to close her eyes and to listen to me carefully, which she does. My sessions scarcely last more than five minutes. I repeat them every day at the same time.

After some days a decided improvement began to manifest itself. After two months of treatment I was able to note the complete disappearance of her nervous fits, headache, nocturnal fears, visual hallucinations, and terrifying dreams. She had a good appetite and ate her meals regularly. One evening, for example, she plucked up her courage and went down into the garden to bring her mother something she had left upstairs, without needing to be accompanied by anyone and without being the least bit frightened. From then on I gradually spaced out the sessions. However, the little girl continued to have learning difficulties, I also counselled against worrying too much about lessons and suggested instead occupying her with housework. Her mother followed this advice.

The little girl occupied herself with work in the house and received only one special lesson every day at home. I saw the child once a week and everything went as well as could be wished. In the month of July it was suggested that the mother let her two children spend four weeks in the country in a sanatorium which took in convalescent or debilitated children for the summer, and where they would be looked after by lay sisters. I advised the mother against letting Eve go. However the child insisted so much that the mother gave in. On the first day of her holiday in the country I received a note from mother with excellent news. Three days later she paid me a visit. The poor woman was in tears, the charitable sister who was looking after Eve had written saying that the little girl was absolutely unable to settle down to her new way of life, that she was homesick and wanted to see her mother, that she wasn't sleeping and was continually agitated etc., and she asked the mother to come and collect the child. I told the mother that the best thing she could do would be to collect the child as soon as possible and bring her to see me immediately.

Six weeks went by before I heard any news. I learnt then that Eve had relapsed into the nervous state she was in originally, and was under the care of another doctor.

It is already more than thirty years since Dr Philips (Durand de Gros) in his remarkable work "Cours de Braidisme" (1860)[77], indicated and called attention to the advantages offered by hypnogogic and suggestive procedures in the treatment of delinquent children:

"Braidism furnishes us with the basis for an intellectual and moral re-education of children which, certainly, will one day be instituted in boarding schools and penitential establishments." (P. 112).

---

[77] *Form of hypnosis associated with the name of James Braid (1795 - 1860).

Dr Liébeault grasped the importance of this and be it "proprio motu"[78] or be it following the guidance of Dr Philips, he put into practice this idea and was able to achieve a good number of cures. After him, Dr Bérillon applied the suggestive method widely in pedagogy, in the treatment of perverse children, and was able to cure a certain number of children presenting with compulsive lying, kleptomania, cruelty, onanism, unremitting laziness, bad behaviour, uncooperativeness and pusillanimity.

Inspired by these examples we have used hypnotic suggestion on many occasions in cases of this type and often, it must be said, this treatment has been shown to be efficacious. We thought we should class the following cases, concerning subjects with hereditary predisposition, in the category Moral Insanity.

## OBS. 52.

MORAL INSANITY, TEMPORARY IMPROVEMENT.

A thirteen-year-old boy, pale, with circles round his eyes, malnourished but well built, is brought to see me by a relative against his will to. He is so frightened that he dare not look at me and tries to hide behind his aunt. Since his tenderest years he was observed to have a leaning towards onanism and not a night went

---

[78] "On his own initiative.

by without him wetting the bed. He is wickedly quarrelsome and lacks all feelings of decency. He likes to be cruel to animals and he lies to excess. He left primary school a year ago and entered the Lycée, where he is not behind in his studies. He is brought to me to be cured of his urinary incontinence, which at the moment is as much diurnal as nocturnal, but also to be cured of his behaviour.

The father, who died three years ago, was an excessively nervous man, the mother is a grand hysteric and completely incapable of controlling her six children. A great disorder reigns in the household. The children haven't the least respect for their mother and are constantly quarrelling amongst themselves.

Persuaded that in order to help this child it would be absolutely necessary to separate him from his environment, I explain to the relative that I am very ready to undertake the treatment of her nephew but on condition that he leaves the maternal roof. The aunt takes on board this change of milieu and asks me insistently to begin the cure straight away.

I succeeded in provoking a deep sleep and had the satisfaction of producing a decided improvement in the patient's condition. The diurnal incontinence disappeared and for several nights afterward he didn't soil his bed. I received good news from his mummy regarding his conduct. In addition I began to have the illusion that I would end up curing this boy notwithstanding the bad milieu in which he continued to live, when one fine day, about three weeks after the beginning of the treatment, I received a visit from his mother telling me that the previous day she had had a frightening scene with her son. I insisted that the lady separate herself from her son and confide him to the care of a family which I designated, letting her know that if she didn't follow my advice I wouldn't be able to continue the treatment. She left me promising to put the necessary arrangements into effect. The next day I saw the patient again with a note from his mother excusing herself and saying that some exceptional reasons had prevented her from keeping her promise. Upon which I gave up the continuing treatment of the boy.

## OBS. 53.

MORAL INSANITY, NOCTURNAL INCONTINENCE OF URINE, VERY MARKED IMPROVEMENT.

A thirteen-year-old boy, seems very healthy, good constitution. He is the only son of a neurasthenic father and a nervous mother. A paternal aunt and a maternal grandmother died mentally ill.

In his early youth the patient contracted whooping cough then measles. At the age of four he had a very severe intestinal disease, at 5 years he had adenoid vegetations scraped in the bucco-pharyngeal cavity. He only ceased to wet the bed at the age of 6. Two years later he had a violent fright at night caused by a fire in the neighbourhood where a woman perished in the flames. Since then he has wet his bed again every night. Reprimanded and punished, his attitude hardened. Instead of improving his condition got worse.

From time to time he deposits faeces in his bed, under furniture, in the corner of his bedroom. He deliberately soils the curtains, the rugs and the drapes with his excrement. He has become a liar, lost all respect for his parents, wants to injure them, dares to threaten them with a knife. He is addicted to masturbation, behaves improperly in the company of children of the opposite sex. He is lazy and won't apply himself.

On the advice of the family doctor the boy was confided to the care of a schoolmaster residing in another village. After two years he returned home, worse than before — with regard to his vices — but having profited a little from primary education.

A specialist in nervous illnesses called in to consult declared the child to be suffering from moral insanity. A treatment suggested by him was followed for some time but didn't have any effect. And so they thought about consulting me.

The boy was brought to me on the 6 January 1893.

Having made an examination, I declared to the parents that I was ready to undertake the treatment of their son on condition that they confide him to the care of an Amsterdam family known to me whom I would tell them about. They were only too happy to hear that I left them some hope of cure and agreed to accede to my request. So I placed the boy with a married teacher, a man of integrity and a good educationalist, who had a small number of residential boys. I began treatment by hypnotic suggestion on 1st January (deep sleep) and repeated the sessions daily until 21 January, from then on I gradually spaced them out. From the 14th of the following April I was no longer hypnotising the bot more than once a week. The result was satisfactory. The nocturnal incontinence only recurred on the 22 January, the 22 February and the 16 March. The boy changed his behaviour, applied himself to his lessons, stopped lying and doing indecent things and became obedient. Everything went well. On the 1 September he was admitted as a pupil in the 6th at the middle school and I continued to have success. However a relapse occurred in January 1894.

The parents had asked me to allow their son to spend his Christmas holidays with them. I gave permission for four days with this restriction, that permission would be withdrawn if I should have complaints about him brought to me before that time. Now on 15 December he happened to piss in his bed and then despite my repeated suggestions the difficulty recurred several times. So I withdrew permission and for a fortnight everything returned to normal. Then the incontinence began again and the teacher reprimanded the boy sharply in front of the other pupils. That incident provoked the patient's anger and was followed by misconduct on his part, such as soiling the walls of the place with excrement.

I had a serious talk with the patient about that. I reminded him that he had been perfectly well behaved for about eleven months and now he was deliberately being naughty. I made him understand that he would end up in a lunatic asylum if he didn't change his behaviour. I spoke to him without the least irritation, I made him feel that I had compassion for him and wanted to help. Eventually he promised me he wouldn't fall back into his bad ways. Upon hearing that, I hypnotised him and repeated my suggestions. From then on I gave him a daily session. The incontinence ceased and his behaviour became once again irreproachable. He left me at the end of July 1894, having been admitted to a special school in order to prepare for an examination, promising to give me news from time to time.

A significant improvement happened in the patient who was the subject of observation 54. The improvement followed psychological treatment so closely and on two occasions that we feel permitted to attribute it to the psychotherapy.

**OBS. 54.**

LYPEMANIA. OBSESSIONAL COMPULSIONS, TEMPORARY IMPROVEMENT.

A worker of medium build, seeming strong and healthy, requests my care on the 31 October 1892. He is a single man aged 36 years and has been working for a long time as a blacksmith and locksmith in his father's business. He has served several masters in the past, however he was never able to stay very long with any of them because of his changeable moods and the variability of his mental state. His father allows him to work only when he feels like it, and lets him take a break as soon as he feels incapable of doing the job.

The patient's mother enjoys good health. The father is taciturn and gloomy. Of his six brothers and sisters none is robust. All are melancholic but most of all his younger sister.

From his earliest days the patient was of a gloomy, withdrawn disposition. At different times he had been unable to do any work for periods of between two and six months. His lypemanic state is accompanied by precordial anxiety and obsessional ideas and compulsions.

*Example 1.* If by chance he touches someone with a bit of leather, he thinks he has poisoned that person. So he tries to convince himself of the ineptitude of the idea by licking the same piece of leather, an action which evidently does him no harm. However the idea that he has poisoned someone continues to obsess him.

*Ex.* 2. When a murder which created a big sensation occurred, he came to believe that he was the murderer and wanted to give himself up to officers of the law.

*Ex.* 3. He is a non-practicing Catholic. However the thought "Prayer will cure you. Go to church", obsesses him.

If he follows that injunction, on leaving the church he feels forced to visit a second and a third church and so on. If he succumbs to the compulsive force, the satisfaction it gives is always incomplete and often non-existent, sometimes he simply becomes even more agitated. Often enough while kneeling in prayer, only sacrilegious words and imprecations come to his mouth. Other times he feels forced to fast, and to confess completely against his will.

In the months of July and August 1874 he spent six weeks in a hospital in Amsterdam from where he was transferred to a hostel for the mentally ill. He left the asylum at the end of the following December. In addition during the course of the year 1888 he underwent an electrical treatment without gaining the least improvement in his state.

Last July (1892) he once again spent about five weeks in hospital where he was treated with hypnotic suggestion. The effect, according to the patient, was negligible. However, in order to get out of the place, he pretended to be cured.

At the present time (31 October 1892) he is extremely agitated. He drags himself from one church to another and finds no respite anywhere, he fears taking his life and at the same time feels impelled toward suicide. He once thought of asking to be readmitted to the hospital he had just left. However he knows that a new stay in that milieu will do him no good. It is that which motivated him to come to me.

All work is repugnant to him, he wanders around town in order to kill time. He takes his meals regularly, eats a lot and with appetite, opens his bowels regularly every day, goes to bed in the evening around ten o'clock and sleeps immediately. The nights are good, he doesn't dream. However at five o'clock in the morning precisely he wakes in a start with the idea: "Get up quickly! Quickly! Go to church!" He eats a quick crust and rushes off to the first mass.

I commenced treatment by suggestion on the same day. I succeeded in giving a bit of peace to my patient who didn't go to sleep but was clearly quite calm during the hour which I set aside for his daily treatment. From the first day he he was able to resist his morning compulsion to go to church, from the third he returned to work in the forge with his father and after a fortnight the improvement was such that he asked my permission to accept a position which had been offered to him of assistant-mechanic on board a steam-ship going from Amsterdam to Mediterranean ports. I gave him that permission. However he didn't follow up on the idea, fearing that his compulsion would overtake him again and that left to his own devices on board and in a foreign country he wouldn't feel strong enough to resist it. He preferred to continue to work with his father.

The patient continued coming to see me every day until the end of March 1893. It is beyond doubt that suggestion did him good and that he was suited to it. The state of psychological depression didn't completely remit, but he told me he no longer had the feeling of despair, the continual agitation and the irresistible compulsions! He was able to continue with his job throughout this time as a perfectly good worker.

I didn't seem again for a period of six weeks. On the 15 May a letter arrived in the post telling me that he had found a well paid job in the Amsterdam area, that everything was going well and that he had to thank me provisionally for my good care.

A fortnight later he came in person. The anxiety had returned and he asked to resume treatment. Calm was again re-established under the influence of suggestion and the patient left me once more restored to good health at the end of the following July. Since then I've had no more news.

Undertaking treatment of chronic melancholia (obs. 55) by suggestion seemed justified to us, since we were convinced that a psychological treatment could only have a beneficial influence. The attempt to create a deep hypnotic state or instead to profit from the period of euphoria that preceded a sleep induced by chloroform, didn't produce the desired results in this case.

### OBS. 55.

CHRONIC MELANCHOLIA, FAILURE OF THE SUGGESTIVE METHOD.

Mrs L. is 62 years old, frail, weak and emaciated, she seems much older. She has been ill for seven years. Before then she enjoyed robust health. She was happily married, she loved her husband and cherished her children who returned her love. She still has five living children who are all now healthy adults, and of whom two are already married.

The illness began with dental caries and persistent headaches. She had all her teeth successively removed, despite which the pains persisted. Different professors and specialists in nervous illnesses, surgeons, renowned dentists in the principal towns of Europe were all consulted to no avail.

Insomnia and excessive irritability followed the pains and gradually evolved into depressive anxiety.

On the advice of a psychiatrist Mrs L. was confined in an asylum where she stayed for three years. Not the least improvement was obtained during that time. So it was decided, above all on the insistence of the patient herself, that she be cared for under the conjugal roof. For about two years Mrs L. had been at home when the doctor treating her suggested to the family a trial of the suggestive method. I was asked to come and see the patient and give my opinion.

*Present state* 24 November 1889.

An excessively thin old lady is sitting in an armchair, indifferent to her surroundings, with dull expressionless eyes, her lip lolling, her mouth half open so that the tip of her tongue is visible. The end of her tongue has a leathery appearance, a consequence of the patient's habit of putting it out all the time and twisting it while screaming or crying.

When I address a word to her she turns slowly toward me after several moments, looks at me and gives correct replies, so long as my questions don't touch on her delusional ideas. She is possessed by the devil, she is cursed, she has killed her husband, she abandoned her children and her husband. She feels an internal fire which slowly burns her. Her stomach is too small to contain everything that people insist that she eats. She cannot walk.

Although obviously weak and asking that she be moved from her bed in a chair, she moves perfectly well of her own accord when she thinks nobody is looking.

She complains of permanent pains in the lower abdomen. On examination I discover nothing abnormal in her abdomen. Every now and again she lets go a shout, complains of infernal pains and accuses herself of imaginary crimes or else she exhausts herself wailing, accusing her nurse of tormenting her and overwhelming the sister with the most vile insults. She no longer suffers with her mouth, the painful tic hasn't appeared for at least five years.

During her stay in the asylum they had recourse to a tube in order to feed her, since then, the threat of tube-feeding again suffices to overcome her resistance if she refuses to eat. However she only ever eats meals against her will. She has often been observed to eat clandestinely when some kind of dish has been left, as if by oversight, in her neighbourhood. Garderobes every morning induced by a warm salt-water enema. Sleep irregular. The patient sometimes sleeps 3 or 4 consecutive hours, sometimes she doesn't sleep at all and spends her night moaning and vociferating, so she often takes quarter or half hour naps during the day.

I didn't have the slightest illusion that suggestion could cure this desperate case, but I wanted to try the method, being convinced that it would do no harm and the possibility existed that I could produce an improvement, especially as the family had insisted that I take on the cure.

The following 6 December I received the patient at home, where she settled into an apartment separate from my house together with one of her daughters and a nurse who had been looking after her for three years.

For the first week I contented myself with observing the patient. I confirmed that in general she slept very little and that her sleep was very irregular. She is often very agitated, sometimes spends more than an hour shouting in a loud voice for no plausible reason while twisting her tongue with her fingers, other times she stays quiet, appears to be occupied with nothing but talks constantly to herself in a low voice. We feed her at fixed times, always under duress, when she breaks out into curses against her nurse. If I come in unexpectedly at a time when she is agitated and is just shouting and moaning, the patient immediately becomes quiet, gathers herself together for a moment and enquires politely after the health of my wife and children. When I ask her: "Would you allow me to treat you?", she always replies that she is damned, that nothing can be done about it, that she cannot be cured; then she invariably repeats the whole series of her delusional ideas.

During the second week I tried to put the patient to sleep every evening at the same time as she went to bed. I made my suggestions slowly, in a low monotonous voice, making simultaneous passes. In that way I succeeded in producing calm and an apparent sleep after about half an hour, when I retired. The first two nights proved to be exceptionally good, on the third night she woke up at 4 o'clock in the morning, the following night she wasn't slow in opening her eyes after my departure and from then on they were just as bad as before.

So on the 15th day I resolved to make an attempt at hypnotism with the aid of chloroform, hoping to be able to take advantage of the excitation phase to make appropriate suggestions. I obtained a deep sleep easily, but I didn't observe the least degree of excitation beforehand. I had only dispensed about 10 ccs. of chloroform. Even so I gave my suggestions of which not one was realised.

The patient slept from 9 o'clock in the evening until 4 o'clock in the morning. On waking she was in a state of anxiety, she had pain in her chest and it was literally impossible to make her eat or drink anything the whole of the following day.

When I came to see her on the evening of the following day she begged me not to make her inhale any more chloroform, because it made her all the worse. I didn't insist, particularly since she was prepared, with a better grace than usual, to comply with my regular procedures in trying to hypnotise her. The night was good and the next day she ate her usual food without resistance.

From then on I continued to give her a hypnotic suggestive session every evening and thus obtained a state of calm and sleep, or apparent sleep, which gradually lengthened with rare exceptions until 6 or 7 o'clock in the morning.

Her general state during the day wasn't in the least changed.

The day of the 30 December was worse than usual. In the evening her anxiety increased. I noted a slight fever, the symptoms of broncho-pneumonia. The next morning the patient presented a non-painful swelling in the right parotid region. The fever increased. Extreme debility. Growing weakness.

During the following days her weakness got worse and worse and between the nights of the 3rd and 4th January the patient expired.

Thus the first epidemic of influenza was spreading in Amsterdam and ravaging the city.

In the following case when suggestion alone was unable to relieve the recurring agitation of a melancholic, the idea came to us — inspired by the excellent results obtained by Dr A. Voisin[79] in the treatment of melancholia by hypodermic injections of morphine — to combine suggestion with morphine injection therapy.

Our hopes of obtaining a deeper hypnotic sleep and thereby augmenting the suggestibility of the patient through the use of morphine were disappointed, and our suggestions achieved nothing more, nor did they prevent habituation to the alkaloid or combat the withdrawal symptoms.

---

[79] Auguste Voisin. Leçons cliniques sur les maladies mentales et les maladies nerveuses. 1883. p. 684 et suivantes.

## OBS. 56.

MELANCHOLIA WITH INSIGHT, MIXED TREATMENT.

A married merchant, aged 60 years, with several cases of mental illness in his family, suffered an attack of melancholia for the first time in 1873, the illness lasted about six months. In 1880 he had a relapse lasting until 1882. He was treated in his own home on each occasion. In spring 1889, premonitory symptoms of a further relapse occurred. Gloomy ideas alternated with a feeling of normal wellbeing. He was very irritable and had attacks of precordial anxiety. The nights were bad. He had a sensation of heaviness at the top of his head. Constipation. Summer and Autumn went by with alternating better and worse periods and the patient continued with his work (book-keeping and overseeing shops) and doing whatever he could.

On the 5 December 1889, the patient accompanied by his wife came to consult me. The previous evening he had been overexcited. Now he is frightened of what he might do to himself, he fears being alone and committing suicide, but above all he fears he might harm his wife. He asks me insistently to watch over him closely, to isolate him and to keep him under surveillance by a very strong man. The family is opposed to the patient being admitted to an asylum and asks me to try hypnotising the patient and treating him by suggestion.

I succeed in putting the patient to sleep and my suggestions do him good and return him to a calm state of mind. That state lasts all day. In the evening at 11 o'clock the patient goes to bed, falls asleep but wakes at 1 o'clock in the morning and cannot get back to sleep.

On the next day 6 December, he comes back to see me. He is agitated. For a second time I manage to produce an obvious sedation, the patient becomes somnolent and realises my suggestion of calm and wellbeing.

I continue the treatment in the following days with gratifying success. However on the 12 December at the time of his appointment the patient is very agitated. His wife tells me that everything was going well and that yesterday evening he began a game of whist enthusiastically, when all of a sudden he threw his cards down and presented the symptoms of a violent agitation. She succeeded in getting him to lie down but he couldn't sleep all night.

I suggest to the family that the patient be taken to my house and be served and looked after by a trusted man. Mrs Z. gladly accepts my proposition but insists on caring for her husband herself as she absolutely doesn't wish to leave him. Around 8 o'clock in the evening Mr. and Mrs Z. took possession of the apartment that I prepared for them. The patient lay down straight away and I managed to put him to sleep after a while. In order to deepen and lengthen the sleep I settled myself at the bedside and spent the whole night next to him. I had the satisfaction of maintaining his sleep by my suggestions until 7 o'clock the following morning. His sleep was troubled by distressing dreams. On awakening the patient was anxious.

Seeing the impossibility of continuing the treatment in this way and persuaded that I wouldn't succeed in curing Mr. Z. by hypnotic suggestion alone, I insisted on consulting the family doctor. That consultation took place and my proposal to combine treatment by suggestion with that of morphine injections as advocated by Dr A. Voisin was agreed by my colleague.

This mixed treatment was followed until 3 April 1890. In fact I succeeded in creating a very satisfactory state in the patient, he slept well, the black ideas bothered him less and he was able to take part in family life. He appeared at the dining table with his wife and shared meals with my family and myself. In the evenings he played his whist or a game of dominoes and occupied himself during the day with writing accounts or drawing. Throughout the last months of his stay with me he took a walk in town every day, either with his wife or with a nurse, and had begun to visit his own house to get himself used to it and to prepare for his return under his own roof. All went well, only we had reached a dose of 200mg. of morphine per day. An attempt on my part to diminish the dose was followed by agitation and delirium which frightened Mrs Z. to such an extent that she lost all confidence and absolutely insisted on interrupting the treatment.

To my great regret Mr Z. left my house several days later for a nursing home in Germany from where he returned cured the following November.

The beneficial effect of suggestion shouldn't be overlooked in observations 57 and 58. In both cases psychological treatment covered all the the medical needs.

## OBS. 57.

MELANCHOLIA WITHOUT DELUSIONS, NOTABLE IMPROVEMENT.

Mr G. was referred to me by a colleague. He is a cigar manufacturer and has known better times. His business had been doing badly for a long time. He is 61 years old, married and no longer has any children at home. Twice in is life he has been through periods of melancholia, at the age of 11 and 23 years. For several months now he has relapsed into melancholia. He has withdrawn into himself, isn't interested in anything, cries all the time and often mutters between his teeth. He spends sleepless nights, dares not set foot outside the house if he isn't accompanied and complains of a sensation of cerebral torpor. He is certain that he no longer understands anything about his business and that he will become impoverished. He feels alone and completely isolated even when in the midst of his family. He gets upset and anxious over nothing. He eats enough but without any appetite. Bowels move regularly.

On the 7 March 1890 he came to consult me for the first time accompanied by a friend. I didn't succeed in putting him to sleep, and so I was confined to prescribing a regime and addressing some calming and encouraging words to him while recommending that he come and see me at the same time on the following day. On the 8 March I obtained the first degree of hypnosis and thanks to my suggestions the patient left me well disposed. Since then I have seen Mr G. every day, gradually the suggested sleep has deepened.

On the following 9 April, the patient's daughter — a primary school teacher — wrote the following lines to me:

" I find that in general my father's state has changed for the better, he doesn't mumble as much as he used to, he's beginning to interest himself in things, he seems less preoccupied.

It is rare now to hear him say: 'I don't understand my business anymore', a phrase which he used to continually reiterate. As before, he is always complaining that business is bad but not without reason. For my part I am sure that if external circumstances were favourable instead of being adverse, as in effect they are, my father would soon be perfectly recovered."

From the beginning of May I gradually spaced out the sessions. The patient now comes to see me alone and he walks at least two hours a day unaccompanied. He has resumed directing work and managing his business. He sleeps regularly every night. It is interesting to study the immediate effect of the suggestions that I give to him. They awaken him, animate him, encourage him. I observe that he repeats my words as and when I pronounce them.

On the 6 November of the same year, another letter was sent to me by Mr G.'s daughter in which she summed up her father's current state in these words: "nothing is wanting from my father's complete recovery witnessed by his own testimony: 'I am better'."

## OBS. 58.

LYPEMANIA, CHRONIC CONSTIPATION, CURE BY HYPNOTIC SUGGESTION.

Mrs L. aged 34 years, married to a labourer, is the mother of four children. Fell ill on the 11 April 1892, she thinks she cannot be cured. She is indifferent to everything, nothing interests her, she only cries and moans all day long. She does the most pressing housework like a veritable robot, however the house shows signs of neglect. Conscientious domestic worker and excellent family mother before her illness, she has become forgetful of her duties, unhappy and melancholic since that time.

Her husband who has only known her happy and content, cherishing her children, no longer recognises her. He remembers having heard it said that around the age of 19, as a young girl, his wife had gone through a period of melancholy in which she ruminated constantly on religious ideas and was obsessed by the question as to whether there was life after death.

Having been informed about the preoccupations of the young girl, the family doctor chastised her harshly and threatened her with being locked up in an asylum if she didn't stop worrying. That threat had an excellent effect and cured her.

In the morning of the 11 April she woke up with a feeling of extreme tiredness accompanied by dizziness. The doctor whom she consulted on the same day reassured her about her condition, telling her that it was quite simply a question of constipation. A purgative that he would prescribe would sort it all out. However the medicine had no effect, the tiredness increased, the patient stayed in bed feeling incapable of doing anything. Another doctor was consulted who diagnosed a nervous breakdown and prescribed some tonics and another purgative. The treatment continued for several weeks and brought about no change in the patient's condition. So a specialist in nervous conditions was consulted, who advised — yet again — laxatives, and recommended that she be admitted to hospital. His advice was followed. On admission to hospital the purgatives were immediately stopped and the patient was submitted to treatment with static electricity and prolonged warm baths. At the end of a month, not feeling the least relief, she left hospital and returned home. A travelling magnetiser then treated her for several days but didn't have the least effect, he advised Mrs L. to consult me.

26 September 1892.

The patient, a small woman with drawn features, thin, unkempt, accompanied by her husband asks me to take her on. She relates the history of her illness in tears, insisting mainly on the fact that she hasn't moved her bowels for six days, that she suffers from persistent constipation and that she would prefer to put an end to her life rather than continue to suffer in this way. The husband tells me that his wife, although unable to do her housework continues to manage as best she can; however she does what she does against her will, just because it is absolutely necessary. She lacks initiative, she pursues and finishes off whatever job he has begun. She is tired all the time. She has never had nervous fits with loss of consciousness, she doesn't like putting things on, making a song and dance like some women (*it's the patient speaking*). She is always sad and depressed. She eats little, sometimes she starts off with appetite but the desire for food immediately leaves her. She doesn't sleep very much. Her periods are normal. On examination there is no pain in the abdomen, it is soft and the colon is full. No hysterical stigmata other than anaesthesia of the whole left hand and the internal part of the forearm on the same side.

I advised Mrs L. to leave all her medicines with me, both internal and external, and to follow my treatment regularly every day. I reassured her about her state of health and promised a certain cure. After having thus been able to calm her anxiety, I succeeded easily in putting her to sleep. She left me after half an hour without any tears and feeling somewhat reassured.

On the third day of treatment she passed hard but copious motions and afterwards a marked improvement became evident.

At the beginning of treatment there was some irregularity of her intestinal function, thus on 7 October the patient was upset by massive bowel movements and diarrhoea, however from the 17 October her visits to the toilet were regular and occurred every day at the same time. The anaesthesia disappeared spontaneously. On the 19 November the patient was entirely recovered, cheerful, healthy, very happy, having become once again a good mother and wife and an excellent housekeeper. I see her again from time to time. No relapses. (September 1894).

With regard to the psychological treatment of chronic alcoholism and dipsomania, we share the ideas of Wetterstrand, Forel and Lloyd Tuckey[80] adumbrated in their publications.

These morbid conditions demand above all a prolonged application of suggestion. With these patients psychological education and support is always de rigueur. We don't mean temporary strategies such as making the drinker sample alcohol while at the same time suggesting that he feels ill, has heart pain or is nauseated by the sight or smell of the drinks from which he will have to withdraw. We prefer to apply ourselves to exercising and reinforcing the will of the individual and to enhancing his psychological state.

Continual attention and care should be paid to keeping alive the sense of responsibility and integrity of individuals. Two difficulties arise here which have to be dealt with. One cannot accord too much liberty to the patient and thus

---

[80] Wetterstrand. Kronick alkoholism, supmani, in: Om Hypnotismens användande i den Praktiska Medicinen. Sid. 40. Stockholm 1888. Ibidem. Om dryckenskapens behandling medelst hypnotisk suggestion. in Hygien. 1888.
Forel. Zur Therapie des Alkoholismus. Münch. Medizin. Wochenschr. No. 26. 1888.
Lloyd Tuckey. The value of hypnotism in chronic alcoholism. London 1892.

expose him to too great a temptation but at the same time one cannot confine him too much and make him feel he is being treated like a child or a prisoner. In overly restricting him the feeling of shame and personal value is weakened and his whole being will gradually tend to recapture its freedom and break its resolutions. This liberation will shine on him like a golden opportunity. Accordingly the first occasion which presents itself will be welcomed with joy and he will use it to go out and paint the town red.

The best tactic to follow and the most preferable is that of letting the patient have the feeling of perfect freedom and autonomy for as long as possible, so that he comes to feel respected by his fellow citizens and develops the illusion that it is his own will which is preventing him from committing excesses.

From the moment that the patient feels the control of another is oppressive, the dangerous sentiment of being in conflict with society is awakened in him with all the subsequent demoralisation. So it is necessary, while remaining constantly on the look out, to preserve the appearance (as long as the patient's misconduct hasn't irreparably damaged it), of dealing with a person who is perfectly together, responsible for his behaviour and on whose word one can rely.

It is impossible to lay down general rules as to the duration of treatment and the quantity of alcohol one can allow the patient.

It is generally believed to be impossible to remove the pernicious hereditary disposition of degenerates which has turned them into alcoholics. Furthermore even the most reliable cure is no lifetime guarantee against a relapse in any patient. In this sense alcoholism or rather the predisposition to alcoholism could be charged with being incurable!

However if a patient without having had recourse to extraordinary means and *vi sua propria*[81] has been able to abstain notwithstanding disadvantageous circumstances for a certain period of time (a year or more) there is room, we believe, to speak of a cure.

To maintain, to consolidate the cure, it is indispensable for the patient — albeit for the rest of his life — to visit the doctor form time to time, perhaps every year. If he doesn't do that, it will cost him a great deal more trouble seek help just when he feels his will is weakening and he needs support.

For the majority of patients complete abstinence from alcoholic beverages is an absolute must. They cannot do better than join a temperance organisation. Membership will

---
[81] * Of their own accord.

smooth out many difficulties and overcome at a stroke numerous little nascent temptations— by having to display them in public — where the patient is averse to being perceived as dishonest.

The wearer of a blue band, a visible sign indicating to everybody that he is a member of an organisation for total abstinence, will be left in peace, and no longer tormented.

In the case of dipsomania an idiosyncrasy for alcohol exists so that a minimal quantity, for example a single glass of house beer, can disturb a person's equilibrium and become the point of departure for much greater excesses.

Only those subjects — well-balanced, but having become alcoholic by habit and through the company they keep — can be permitted to continue drinking a certain quantity of wine or beer.

No need to recall here a well known vice of drinkers, above all the less intelligent — the penchant for lying. They love to cover up their excesses or represent them as insignificant breeches of the prescribed regime.

These patients are for the most part very suggestible.

## OBS. 59.

PERIODIC DIPSOMANIA, CURE BY HYPNOTIC SUGGESTION. RELAPSE.

Mrs B. is 36 years old and has always been a nervous person. Her mother and two other sisters suffered with nervous fits of a hysterical kind.

Married at the age of 23, she gave birth the following year to a boy who is still alive. That boy is now twelve years old and has inherited the nervous disposition of his mother. Five years ago, a second pregnancy was followed by the birth of a child who died after three weeks. Severely ill during and after the births, it took a long time for her to recover her strength. On the advice of her doctor, while convalescing, she began to drink cognac and English beer. The beginning of her dipsomania dates from that time. During or after her periods she felt the need to drink beer, wine, liqueurs, in short anything she could get her hands on. At first the drinking bouts scarcely lasted longer than 3 or 4 days, but latterly they have often lasted 13 to 15 days. They begin with a ringing in her ears. Without feeling thirst or any marked desire for spirits she feels an irresistible, obsessive desire to get drunk. Once she is in that state she is horrible, hurls abuse at her husband or child or whoever opposes her mania for drink, she acts like a crazy person and is immune to all notions of modesty. After the crisis, a huge tiredness overcomes her, she hides herself from view and is full of remorse, makes promises that she will never keep, goes about her housekeeping again and becomes sober.

Everything has been tried, the advice of different doctors has been followed, she was admitted to a mental hospital for three months, all without useful results. For tow years the husband has cherished the inappropriate idea of buying and running a cafe-restaurant, something singularly favourable the destructive leanings of his wife.

A friend of the husband recommended that his wife be treated with hypnotic suggestion. The lady, having agreed to a trial of treatment, came to see me for the first time on 6 March 1893.

The patient had to make a two hour train journey. While talking, her breath betrayed the fact that she had not yet taken a vow of sobriety.

She admitted having drunk during the previous day. She had been abstinent from that evening, furthermore she was coming to the end of a drinking bout. She assured me that she really wanted to be rid of the awful habit but she didn't know how, being unable to resist her obsessive desire.

I promised to try to give her the will power and strength to resist her unhealthy leaning. An attempt to put her to sleep failed, she didn't sleep, seemed unaffected by my words, however she remained lying down on a chaise longue, eyes closed, for almost an hour and left me with the promise of abstaining completely from alcoholic drinks.

The next phase occurred probably towards the middle of the following March.

13 March, 2nd session. Light sleep that I prolonged for two hours.

20 March, 3rd session. Her periods have been on for four days. The patient hasn't had any ringing in her ears, hasn't felt the need to drink.

27 March, 4th session. Menstruation only stopped yesterday. She has never had a period for such a long time. All is well.

11 April, 5th session. Continues to keep well.

24 April, 6th session. Her period started on the 16 and the loss finished on the 21. Everything is going well. The husband is all over himself with thanks in his letters.

5 June, 7th session.

Menstruation occurred on 26 May without incident. Continues to be well. I allow the patient to defer her next visit for two months.

On the 24 August her husband tells me that his wife refused to come to my session on the 5 August, that she kept well until two days ago. She is having a period, she has had a relapse.

A letter which I addressed to the poor woman requesting her insistently to resume her treatment, has been left without a response.

## OBS. 60.

PERIODIC DIPSOMANIA. CURE LASTING THREE YEARS. RELAPSE.

Mr A. aged 37 years is a dipsomaniac and habitual drinker. He presents bouts of irresistible drinking. When the desire takes hold of him, at first he feels run down and ill, feels like vomiting, then he gives way to greater excesses. Apart from these binges he is a habitual drinker, he drinks in smaller quantities and is so adept at hiding his vice that nobody in his family has noticed it.

He has been admitted to a nursing home several times for a rest cure; every time withdrawal symptoms immediately appear and thus reveal to the doctor, the alcohol abuse to which the patient is addicted and which he has omitted to confess.

The patient seems healthy, he is well built and enjoys an excellent constitution, however he shows the psychological stigmata of degeneracy. Apart from his dipsomania, he has an exaggerated sexual appetite which he indulges rampantly. He is aware of often feeling an overwhelming need to lie to and cheat the people around him. He is debauched. He was married, became a father to two children and then a widower, his family found themselves having to declare him incapable in order to place him under guardianship and gain control over his money and belongings.

Admission to a sanatorium is the only effective way of preventing his excesses. Indeed from time to time he stays there for several months at a time. If left to his own devices, he pretends to be abstinent for a long time but continues to drink clandestinely until at a given moment he can no longer hide his behaviour.

The patient presents himself very well and knows how to affect the manners of a well-bred man, on whom one can absolutely rely.

In March 1890 he requested my care and I instituted treatment by suggestion.

From the first session, my suggestions took hold of him, and in so far as it has been possible to observe the patient, he has been abstinent from the least excess for three consecutive years. At first I gave daily sessions then I continued them at greater intervals. He joined a total temperance organisation, moved about Amsterdam freely and spent his time agreeably doing light work.

If he wasn't binging during this period, it seemed however that he also wasn't leading a chaste life, and his debauched leanings made a mockery of my suggestions.

The lack of any withdrawal symptoms during a voluntary in-patient stay in his usual sanatorium, during the three year period, leant weight to the supposition that he had indeed kept his promise of temperance.

At the beginning of the year 1893 he suffered an acute attack of rheumatism which forced him to stay at home for several weeks. From that time he gradually evaded my influence, he put an end to his regular visits and reverted to his bad habits above all of a sexual and debauched kind, which necessitated admission to a nursing home.

However although he was never seen in a state of inebriation during this period, the debts which he ran up suggested that in this regard as well, he hadn't kept his promise of sobriety.

As he was pretending to continue his treatment with me but was in fact doing nothing — which we eventually became aware of — it was impossible to allow him to continue to be master of his own actions and he had to be readmitted.

The salutary effect of suggestion lasting three years was perhaps misunderstood, but from the moment that certain circumstances undermined his regular treatment, the fight became unequal for the patient and the relapse imposed itself.

## OBS. 61.

ALCOHOLISM CURED BY SUGGESTION.

An 18-year-old adolescent, stocky, well built, strong, was born of parents who were exempt from nervous problems. Of his twelve brothers and sisters several suffer from nerves, two sisters are grand hysterics.

He received a harsh education and never left his town of birth, nor his parents guardianship, when at the age of 17 he found himself living on his own in a furnished apartment in Amsterdam, in order to attend special lessons and prepare for an examination. Dragged along by some comrades who led the high life, he developed a taste for drink and became habitually drunk.

His father's remonstrances and threats had no effect. Notwithstanding his promises to correct his ways, he succumbed to temptation again every time.

One of his sisters (a grand hysteric), one of my old patients, brought him to me one day and asked me to look after the wayward boy.

I had the satisfaction of immersing him in a deep sleep at the first attempt at hypnotism, and I made use of it to suggest a disgust for strong drink while at the same time permitting him one or two glasses of beer per day.

I saw the patient again after eight days, he had abstained from strong drink but he confessed to having drunk six glasses of very alcoholic beer the previous day which had made him drunk.

I put him to sleep again and repeated my previous suggestion, this time forbidding beer as well.

Having learnt that his father wanted him to join the army, I spoke to him about it before putting him to sleep. He wasn't keen on the idea, however I inspired him — thanks to an appropriate hypnotic suggestion — with such a love of the service that after a few days he enrolled.

Since then I have seen him again on two occasions, widely spaced. He has become and remains sober, a result probably due in part to the severe discipline of the regiment, but doubtless also partly due to my suggestions.

He has served two years in the army now and his conduct seems to be exemplary.

## OBS. 62.

ALCOHOLIC HABITS. CURE.

Mr W. abuses alcoholic drinks on a daily basis, he is 35 years old and is in a respectable position. In his family drunkeness is a common enough fault. To be honest, the patient's father makes wide use of fermented drinks without falling into drunkenness.

The patient spent some time in Germany as a student. While he was there he contracted the habit of drinking a lot of beer. It was only later, however, after marrying and achieving a good social position, that he fell into excesses that threatened his career and disturbed his peace at home. Mr W. had already been leading an unruly life for ten years when he came to consult me for the first time. He wasted his money and drank all sorts of alcoholic drinks but mostly a lot of beer. If he came across setbacks or problems he fell into such excesses that his wife had all the difficulty in the world in preventing misfortunes. Otherwise he is a mild mannered, loving man who cherishes his wife,

I began his treatment in April 1891. He seemed quite healthy, perfectly fit and didn't reveal any nervous symptoms or stigmata of degeneration, but he had a weak character, too malleable. He couldn't remember having spent a single day without getting drunk since he was a student.

With regard to alcoholic drinks, I allowed him to drink a bottle of beer every day and to keep it at that.

My suggestions of sobriety took effect and the patient was holding up well until September 1893. At first I gave him one session per week, then I treated him at greater intervals, finally I only saw him from time to time, when he felt his will was weakening. Towards the end of 1893 he neglected coming to see me, and with the aid of setbacks and bad friends, he forgot his promises two or three times and overindulged. Happily he came back in time to resume his treatment. I reduced his permitted ration of alcoholic drink to half a bottle of barley beer per day. So far he has not relapsed. He continues to see me once a month. His wife has expressed her gratitude many times for the good I have done her husband, leading to the restoration of peace in the household.

———————

## A. GROUP IV.

### Neuropathic conditions.

Nothing is more striking and more persuasive for a beginner in psycho-therapy than to see the calm established by suggestion in an attack of asthma. Years ago, when I was still involved in my first trials of hypnotism, I had the good luck to be looking after a lady aged about 70, nephritic and troubled to the highest degree by asthma attacks.

I remember very well one day, called in haste to give her an injection of morphine, which was the only thing that relieved her, I arrived and found the supply of morphine exhausted. Her respiratory distress was very great, the time necessary to get hold of the medication was about half an hour. I suggested to the patient that I put her to sleep and relieve her by suggestion. She agreed and I wasn't a little astonished to observe sleep come over her after a few passes and calming words. I suggested the disappearance of her symptoms with some hesitation at first, then with boldness and growing conviction. In less than five minutes the attack was totally arrested and the patient continued to sleep calmly and peacefully. Needless to add that from then on for this lady, suggestion continued to replace injections.

We are of the opinion that in nervous asthma, hypnotic suggestion constitutes the remedy par excellence and that its employment is also indicated as an agent of symptomatic and palliative relief in other varieties of asthma.

We share the opinion of Dr Brugelmann[82]: "that we have the right, that it is our duty, to suggest the cure, even in doubtful cases!"

We never have to fear harming the patient if in order to combat the symptom we resort to suggestion.

## OBS. 63.

BRONCHIAL ASTHMA, CURE BY HYPNOTIC SUGGESTION.

Mr H. lost his parents at a very young age. His father died of a heart condition, his mother was a very nervous woman. At the age of 16½ he volunteered for service in a company of sappers. However the service was too demanding for him, so one fine morning — after having done many fatigues the previous day — he woke up with a sensation of suffocation. He was having his first attack of asthma. He was coming up to his 18th birthday. Since then these attacks have increased. He continued his service, which included several stays in a military hospital, until he was discharged in the month of November 1888. After being acquitted from military service he hadn't any asthmatic symptoms for about

---

[82] Conf. Psycho-therapie und Asthma von Dr. W. Brugelmann in Peitsch. f. Hypnot. von Dr. Grossman. Januar 1894. S. 107.

six months. But a catarrhal infection gained him a renewed attack of asthma which from that time on has often recurred. The treatment which he has followed consists of the administration of potassium iodide in high doses during the intervals and morphine injections during the attacks. His last attack dates from six weeks ago and lasted about 48 hours.

*Present state* 9 January 1891.

A man of average build, appearing quite healthy, asks me to rid him by hypnotic suggestion of vague pains in the left hip, in the right shoulder and in the front of his thorax. He had a bad night due to these pains. He's coming to me because he thinks he is a neuropath and the medicine he has been prescribed (salicylates) makes him ill. On questioning, he lets me know that he suffers from intermittent attacks of asthma. These attacks ordinarily come in the wake of either intellectual or physical overwork. Certain fumes, those of new rubbery objects, those emanating from asphalt melted by heat or a peat fire, various emotions, a coryza or bronchial catarrh, can provoke an attack. He has become so susceptible that he avoids going out as much as possible and for several months he has felt unable to go to his office. He has had to give up his employment as a book keeper in a shop. He feeds himself well, eats with appetite, isn't constipated. He sleeps well if he doesn't have any pains and if he is breathing freely.

On examination I note that nothing in his lungs, heart or nose explains the asthma attacks.

I succeed in putting the patient to sleep without any difficulty and in ridding him of his pains. After repeating my sessions during the following days, the pains disappeared for good and the patient learnt to give up his normal housebound state. He plucked up his courage, went out every day, took walks that he gradually prolonged and after a fortnight was in a good enough condition to resume his clerical employment.

Having got to this stage I gave him sessions at intervals of three to four days.

During the night of 21 to 22 January the patient was surprised by an asthma attack accompanied by febrile symptoms (T. 38.4°C.) The attack resolved itself on the evening of the 22. He came to see me in the afternoon of the 23. His respiration was perfectly free, nothing seemed amiss by then. I resumed the sessions on a daily basis and continued them for the following 15 days, then I gradually spaced them out more and more. The last session dated 3 June. He had no more attacks after the 22 January.

On the following 13 August, the patient who had left Amsterdam for a provincial town where he found a good job, wrote to me that all was well, his health left nothing to be desired and the asthma had not reappeared.

On the 25 January 1894, thus three years after the beginning of the suggestive treatment, Mr H. whom I had asked for news, replied that if during the early stages of his stay in the provinces he still had a little difficulty in breathing, he could assure me that his heath now — thanks to my suggestions — left nothing to be desired. He couldn't remember having had a severe asthma attack since he left Amsterdam, so he considered himself completely cured.

## OBS. 64.

BRONCHIAL ASTHMA, DECIDED IMPROVEMENT.

W. d. V. is 22 years old. He is a medical student, son of a neurasthenic father and a nervous mother. The grandfather and a maternal aunt died mentally ill. This young man suffered nervous asthma attacks at the age of 18 months after the disappearance of an *impetigo* on his face. Since then he has never been rid of them. At the age of 19 years he had an attack of croupous pneumonia from which he is perfectly recovered.

He has undergone different treatments. For two years he had quarterizations of his nasal mucosa. Arsenic, belladonna and potassium iodide, were the mainstays of the treatment in their turn. He followed a compressed-air treatment for a long time, finally he spent some time on the island of Madeira. All these treatments appeared salutary at the beginning and all of them failed in the end.

On 13 January 1893, the patient came to consult me for the first time in the midst of an attack.

I succeeded in putting him to sleep and making the asthmatic syndrome disappear completely by suggestion. The dyspnoea[83] resolved with an evacuation of sputum after about an hour. So I

---

[83] * Breathlessness.

woke up the patient who felt he had been asleep but remembered perfectly everything I had said and done. In the morning of the 15 January, thus the day after next, an immediately aborted attack occurred. At the time of his session, notably 11.30am, his respiration was entirely free. Mr.d.V followed my treatment assiduously, at first daily, then at longer and longer intervals.

He continued with his studies and flattered himself that he was already clear of his illness when on the following 6 August in the morning, he woke up in the middle of an attack. At that time he was in the provinces where he was taking a few days holiday. The attack was preceded and precipitated by a bronchial catarrh. When the patient returned to see me, the neurosis had regained control of him and resisted my suggestions for several days. It was only after a fortnight that Mr d.V felt completely recovered. It is fair to say that the relapse coincided with a strong emotion that the patient experienced, notably with a goodbye visit made by his only brother who at the time was leaving for Brazil, pursuing a course that would keep him in America for several years.

I am continuing the treatment. The patient comes to see me twice a week. He has remained free of his neurosis up till now. (February 1894).

## OBS. 65.

PERIODIC BRONCHIAL ASTHMA, HEMICRANIA. CURE OF THE ASTHMA, NOTABLE IMPROVEMENT OF THE MIGRAINE.

A married lady, aged 41 years had been subject to asthma attacks for several years coming fairly regularly every evening at the same time and lasting deep into the night. Quinine, arsenic, potassium iodide had been tried in vain.

In recent times she has warded off attacks by burning nitrated paper and inhaling the fumes. She only succeeds in sleeping if she has burned her paper.

She also suffers from migraine. Attacks often occur, sometimes twice a week, following some kind of overwork, or changes in her usual routine, when she is forced to stay in bed for 12 to 36 hours. Most often the attacks finish with vomiting sputum and bile. She avoids going to shows and concerts and going out into the world as much as possible, because she knows that her headache will not fail to appear the moment that she gets ready to go out.

The patient has no organic lesions which could account for her syndromes. There is a family history of nervous conditions. Although the patient herself is absolutely exempt from hysterical stigmata, some of her sisters and her mother have presented symptoms of a hysterical and neurasthenic kind.

I observed and treated this lady with suggestion often at intervals of several months and I succeeded in absolutely ridding her of her asthma, and reducing the attacks of migraine to a minimum frequency and intensity. It will soon be nearly four years since she has had an attack of breathlessness and the migraine leaves her periods of respite lasting three to ten months consecutively.

In hypnotising this lady I only ever succeeded in obtaining a light sleep.

Hey fever, a condition often tenacious and resistant to a number of medicines can easily be treated by suggestion.

### OBS. 66.

ASTHMATIC HEY FEVER, CURE BY HYPNOTIC SUGGESTION.

On the 4 June 1890 I received a visit from a 52-year-old man subject to asthmatic hey fever. For almost twenty years he had been troubled every year by this illness which lasted at least six weeks. He had tried everything to cure it but no treatment had worked for him.

Otherwise he enjoys good health, he is never ill.

The asthma took hold of him this year on the 26 of last May. He described his condition as follows: "As soon as I wake up in the morning I feel my eyelids are swollen and sticky and begin to sneeze. I sneeze continually till just before the afternoon or towards evening, and I produce a lot of mucous from my nose and mouth. It's only around 5.30pm that I manage to eat anything, immediately after taking a rest I go to sleep and only wake up around 9 o'clock with a stuffy sensation. So I want, I feel the need to cough but I can't, my breathing becomes more and more difficult and an asthma attack gradually develops. The asthma lasts till midnight and often even until 3am, that is to say until I succeed in getting to sleep. On waking I begin to sneeze again and so it goes on."

I treated the patient on the 4, 5, 7, 9, 13, and 15 June. From the first session I succeeded in breaking the morbid concatenation, suppressing the sneezing and procuring an excellent night for the patient without asthma.

The hypnotic sleep provoked was deep, the patient was very suggestible. From the fifth session he was cured and nothing more occurred.

## OBS. 67.

ASTHMATIC HEY FEVER, NOTABLE IMPROVEMENT.

27 August 1889. First consultation. The patient has been subject to hey fever for more than 30 years. The asthma happens every summer and becomes so severe that the patient sometimes finds himself condemned to remain sitting in an armchair for several days in a row without being able to get undressed or lie down. The attack is heralded by irritability of the nasopharyngeal mucosa and sneezing accompanied by some difficulty in breathing. That sensation of difficulty occurs mainly during the night and morning and gradually develops into a full blown asthma attack. The

syndrome lasts at least three or four weeks and ends with a persistent cough and the expectoration of phlegm.

The patient has not been exempt from asthma for a single year. However a stay in a mountainous country on a high-plateau seemed to decrease and shorten the attacks.

Mr B. is a thin elderly man, short but well built. He ordinarily enjoys excellent health. On examination I am able to note the absence of emphysema, bronchitis, anatomical lesions of the heart, and nasal conditions.

We advised the patient to come and see us later on towards the end of next May.

On the 17 May 1890 Mr B. came for the second time. He was in good health, had no premonitory asthmatic symptoms.

When hypnotised he reaches the second degree of sleep. No amnesia.

In spite of my suggestions, the initial symptoms: sneezing, increased irritability of the nasopharyngeal mucosa, the beginning of difficulty in breathing, occurred on the third day of treatment. However the difficulty in breathing disappeared completely under hypnosis after an appropriate suggestion.

The patient's condition is very satisfactory, notably shortness of breath begins to occur occasionally but is immediately brought to an end by a suggestion. The patient, believing he was in a risky area, left town for his residence in the country on the 15 of the following June. Scarcely had he got on the train than he was overcome by an attack, and on arrival at his country home he was suffocating. For eight days it was literally impossible for him to move out of his armchair. A slight remission of symptoms occurred and he made the return journey to Amsterdam, and came back to see me on the 28 June. Thanks to hypnotic suggestion all respiratory difficulties soon disappeared. The patient remained under my care for another three weeks, "swearing, but a little late, that the asthma would never take hold of him again."

The patient took better measures in the years 1891 and 1892. He spent the risky time in my clinic and remained free from his asthma. A small amount of sneezing at the beginning and a catarrhal cough and the end of his stay constituted the only troubles that the patient suffered.

## OBS. 68.

ASTHMATIC HEY FEVER, CURE.

Mrs K. v. D. is 72 years old. She consults me in March 1893, informing me that since 1847 she has been subject to asthmatic hey fever virtually every year as summer approaches.

The exceptions, that is to say the years when she hasn't been disturbed by this neurosis, were those that she spent in the Indies or near the sea on the crossing. During the other years, her infirmity rendered her sick for at least six weeks, with sneezing, asthma and an accompanying state of general malaise and fever constituting the principal symptoms. Mrs K. v. D. is a robustly healthy lady and has no organic lesions of her thoracic organs.

No treatment has done her any good nor has any been able to shorten the duration of the syndrome.

I asked the patient to come and see me on the 15 of the following May.

On that date I began treatment by hypnotic suggestion. Light but satisfactory hypnosis producing a state of pronounced calm. No sign of prodromal symptoms was produced. I succeeded through an extended treatment lasting six weeks (daily sessions at a fixed time lasting about an hour) in warding off the illness. Indeed Mrs K. v. D. contrary to her enforced seclusion during the fateful period, has been able to follow her usual daily life. She goes out every day, takes her accustomed walk, comes to see me at the clinic and can pursue her usual occupations. Some indications of irritation of the pituitary mucosa and of difficulty in respiration, immediately suppressed by appropriate suggestion, present momentarily from time to time.

The patient felt no joy at having been relieved of her annual torment in such an agreeable and commodious manner and intends to demand the same treatment next year.

The treatment of stutterers by hypnotism was particularly recommended by Wetterstrand. In his book cited several times, he reports 48 treated cases of which he cured 15. Doctor Ringier in his excellent work[84] is less enthusiastic.

---

[84] Erfolge des Therapeut. Hypnotismus in der Landpraxis. 1891.

Out of ten treated cases he was only able to obtain two cures and three marked improvements followed by relapses.

Like him, we are of the opinion that it is very difficult to cure stuttering by hypnotism alone. Conscious or unconscious auto-suggestion plays a preponderant role in maintaining the syndrome.

If one fails to succeed in putting the patient into a deep sleep, direct suggestion will be of scarcely any use, and one will be forced to suggest the gradual disappearance of the patient's general state of nerves and to exercise the faculty of speech systematically during and after hypnosis.

## OBS. 69.

RECENT ONSET OF STUTTERING IN A BOY, CURED BY HYPNOTIC SUGGESTION.

A 13-year-old boy, son of a father who was a stutterer in his youth but who had been able to overcome his defect and a mother who had been mentally ill for a long time, he had never had the least difficulty in speaking correctly until two months earlier. He was at school and was told by the master to read a fable out loud to the class. It was the first time for him, and the emotion triggered his stuttering. He hasn't been able to get rid of it since then. On consulting the family doctor, the young man was advised to come and see me.

I succeeded in getting him into a deep sleep in the first session. But although the patient was very suggestible, it took several sessions to get him to speak and recite during sleep, without stuttering. Once this result was obtained, I was soon able to get him to overcome his speech defect in a waking state.

After a fortnight I had won my case, in fact not only was the boy no longer stuttering but he had achieved a state of calm and poise which he previously lacked.

After that I saw him again three or four times at increasing intervals and more than a year later I had news confirming his cure.

**OBS. 70.**

STUTTERING AND SPASMODIC FACIAL TIC, VERY MARKED IMPROVEMENT, CONTINUATION OF TREATMENT.

The younger son of a country doctor, a 14-year-old boy, stuttered from his early infancy. The father is neurasthenic, the mother is a bit hysterical. The boy seems well built, he is big for his age. He is nervous, short tempered and it seems to me not very obedient to his parents. He has a habit of speaking quickly, of expressing himself volubly, he stammers and soon becomes incapable of articulating a word. The efforts he makes in order to overcome the difficulty, accompanied by a spasmodic facial tic, only worsen his speech defect. He is a bad pupil, doesn't apply himself. Expected to go to military school, his father fears he will be rejected from the service because of his infirmity.

The patient was plunged into a deep sleep from the first session. On waking he read a newspaper article I gave him faultlessly and without hesitation.

I treated the boy for a fortnight and I inculcated a state of calm during his sleep, predicting that on waking he would no longer have the least difficulty in speaking, that he would no longer stutter, that he would no longer make those hideous grimaces whilst speaking; from the moment that he stopped being agitated and applied himself to speaking slowly.

I sent him back home afterwards and only saw him again twice a month. He continued to speak without difficulty, he was hugely calmer and applying himself much more at school.

At rare moments when his self-possession lapsed, the stuttering immediately reappeared. I am continuing the treatment and have no doubt that a complete cure will be obtained.

We have often had occasion to treat chronic intestinal constipation resistant to all medicines. In the four cases which presented in isolation that is to say the patients had no associated conditions, we obtained one cure, one very marked improvement, one no effect; and finally a patient who provided us with no further news after his first session. Constipation generally goes along with all sorts of other symptoms presented by our patients and it has to be said that suggestion often succeeds, where purges and enemas come to nothing.

We urge our colleagues to read Professor Forel's article: "The cure of constipation by suggestion"[85], which is very instructive on this subject.

The results obtained in the treatment of chorea strongly suggest recourse to psycho-therapy in cases of this type. Different authors, notably Liébeault, Bernheim, Wetterstrand, Dumontpalier, to say nothing of others, have published the most convincing observations.

Similarly cures of onanism are no less remarkable. Often suggestion, even without prior sleep, succeeds in curing inveterate cases resistant to all other treatments. Bernheim's, Bérillon's, Liébault's and von Schrenk-Notzing's publications — and passing on from the finest, our own — lend weight to our assertions.

### OBS. 71.

HABITUAL MASTURBATION; IMPROVEMENT.

A young man aged 27 years confessed to me that he had been addicted to onanism since the age of 13, nearly every day. He lives in a small provincial town where there is little opportunity of

---

[85] Zeitschrift für Hypnotismus Nov. 1893.

seeing a girl, also he has never cohabited. He remembers having gone fifteen days without masturbating during the course of an illness.

His father died of cancer of the stomach. His mother, a very nervous woman, is still alive. He lives with his mother and a sickly aunt. He hasn't had any serious illnesses. He underwent primary and secondary education in the town where he lives.

He gets up at 9.30am, goes to bed at 11o'clock in the evening and masturbates before going to sleep. He eats very well and doesn't drink to excess. He doesn't like outdoor exercise or walks, he doesn't go out much, doesn't see many people, likes to be alone but doesn't shun society. Doesn't complain of tiredness, pains or anxiety. His memory is excellent, he is inclined to study, avoids erotic reading. He is annoyed at being addicted to onanism, knows that it ruins his health and hopes that suggestion will be able to free him of this bad habit.

He doesn't seem to be suffering, he has a pale yellowish complexion and is slightly timid.

I undertook treatment on 5 February 1893. I prescribed him a regimen and suggested that he would have the strength to resist his bad habit. The hypnosis obtained didn't exceed a state of somnolence. The treatment continued until the following 3 October. I gave twelve sessions in all. During this time the patient gave way to temptation twice, on the 13 July and the 15 August. Unexpected circumstances gave him cause to interrupt the treatment. The patient confirmed that he felt able to resist all temptation and that he had fully recovered his will power.

He assured me that he would definitely come back to see me if he ever fell back into his habit.

A single observation of paralysis agitans[86] in which the effect obtained by suggestion was dubious is insufficient to make a judgement as to its value. Let us remember that Doctor Luys reported several cures of this disease obtained by the use of a rotating mirror.

On the other hand, we can judge the value of psychotherapy in urinary incontinence with more authority.

### OBS. 72.

DIURNAL AND NOCTURNAL INCONTINENCE OF URINE. PERIODIC CEPHALGIA. CURE.

A 12-year-old boy, well built, strong for his age. Very much nervous illness in his family history. Suffers periodic cephalgia. Often urinates in bed. During the day the need is sometimes so urgent that he hasn't time to get anywhere. I treated him with suggestion from October 1888 to April 1889. From February 1889 he stopped soiling his underwear during the day and the nocturnal incontinence only occurred at two or three weekly intervals. He came to see me one more time in June 1889 and told me that it

---

[86] **Parkinson's disease.**

hadn't happened for six weeks. He left Amsterdam and only came back a year later. He told me then that he was completely free of incontinence and only disturbed by his headaches from time to time at widely spaced intervals.

## OBS. 73.

NOCTURNAL INCONTINENCE OF URINE, CURE.

A young man aged 17 years. Serious nervous family history. Urinary incontinence almost every night. Treated with suggestion from June 1888 to July 1889. Improvement so that his accident occurred no more than once or twice a month. He came to see me for the last time in September 1889, intending to leave Holland and go abroad.

On the 20 February 1893 he returned from his travels, came to see me and told me that for the first year after his departure, the accidents were still happening about once every six or or eight weeks. During the following year he was completely rid of his difficulty. A final and sole episode of incontinence occurred in February 1891. After leaving Amsterdam, he hadn't had any more treatment.

## OBS. 74.

URINARY INCONTINENCE, CURED BY HYPNOTIC SUGGESTION, RELAPSE FOLLOWED BY DEFINITIVE CURE.

A malnourished, nervous, weakly boy, having been cured of incontinence by suggestion in June 1889, requested my care in the following December for a relapse of his problem. A single suggestion during a state of deep sleep sufficed to suppress the problem for good. The cure has not yet been belied.

## OBS. 75.

URINARY INCONTINENCE, CURE.

A young girl aged 14 years, robust constitution, excellent health. Minor family history of nervous conditions. Not yet having periods. Involuntary nocturnal emission. Sometimes she has an accident over a series of nights, sometimes a fortnight can pass without anything happening. Was treated for six weeks in 1889. Light hypnotic sleep. At that time the incontinence happened on two occasions. The patient being unable to prolong her stay, the treatment was interrupted.

During the course of the years 1890 and 1891 she came to see me intermittently at one or two monthly intervals. The result was excellent since afterwards the accident only occurred on rare occasions and disappeared completely from 21 October 1891. Up till now (February 1894) the cure has lasted.

## OBS. 76.

NOCTURNAL INCONTINENCE OF URINE, FAILURE.

An orphan girl aged 16 years, seamstress, daughter of a mother who died mentally ill and a drunken father, has peed in her bed from earliest infancy and has continued to do so every night. She is in the care of an aunt who would very much like to be relieved of her niece. She is brought to my consultation against her will. She presents no organic lesions or hysterical stigmata.

My attempts to hypnotise her do not succeed in the face of the bad will manifested by the patient. After several unproductive sessions, I didn't see her again.

## OBS. 77.

NOCTURNAL INCONTINENCE OF URINE, CURE.

A young peasant girl, aged 17 years, perfectly developed and of robust appearance, very timid, no family history of nerves and having no organic lesions, is subject to nocturnal urinary incontinence.

Few nights go past when she doesn't pee in her bed. The village doctor has declared her incurable.

First consultation: 16 September 1889. As she lives a long way from town it is difficult for her to come for treatment more than twice a week. From the fourth session she went into a deep sleep.

Treatment by suggestion was continued until 10 September 1890. Thus, during that year she had 27 sessions at gradually increasing intervals. Her condition gradually improved. During the last six months the problem only occurred six times. Special circumstances forced my patient to abandon the treatment prematurely. In December 1892 I received a visit from her mother who informed me that her daughter had not been peeing in her bed for the last six months. Since my last session the incontinence had occasionally happened but infrequently.

## OBS. 78.

NOCTURNAL INCONTINENCE OF URINE, TREATMENT BY HYPNOTIC SUGGESTION, RESULT UNKNOWN.

A little girl, ten years old, scrofulous, thin, malnourished, was brought to see me by her mother, a Polish Jewish lady.

This lady tells me (in the German language) that her child sleeps very deeply and pees in bed every night. She asks me to rid her little girl of this unfortunate habit.

The child only understands Polish, a language which is completely foreign to me. Schooled by the mother, who translated some German phrases for me into Polish, I try to make my suggestions as well as I can in the child's idiom. The little girl falls into a deep sleep and I have some difficulty in waking her. At intervals of three to four days I gave five sessions to my little

Polish girl. Her condition improved markedly. As I have not seen her again nor had any news I don't know the definitive result.

## OBS. 79.

NOCTURNAL INCONTINENCE OF URINE, CURE.

A robust young man, well built, aged 17 years, without any family history of nerves. Is a little retiring. Little aptitude for his studies. Pees in bed two or three times a week. No organic lesions. I suspect him of being addicted to masturbation.

I treated this boy for two years. During that time I gave him twenty sessions of suggestion in a state of deep sleep with intervals at first of two or three days, then three weeks to six months. During those two years incontinence occurred eleven times. Since the 14 December 1892 the cure has been maintained. The latest news dates from January 1894.

## OBS. 80.

CHRONIC NOCTURNAL INCONTINENCE OF URINE, CURE.

A 17-year-old young man, weak, debilitated, very nervous, with a serious family history of nerves, referred to me by the family doctor. He pees in bed every night. The operation of phimosis has been carried out without bringing any happy modification of the bad habit. The doctor has tried the usual drugs without result and asks me to undertake a treatment by hypnotic suggestion.

The first session given in the presence of the doctor on 22 August 1891 resulted in the patient having no further involuntary emissions before the following 10 September. The second session took place on the 19 September and the patient remained exempt from his problem for three weeks.

From then on I continued to give my sessions at intervals of between two to six weeks until the middle of August 1893.

From time to time the incontinence occurred during those two years, in all about twelve times. On his last visit (Sept. 1894) the difficulty hadn't appeared for thirteen months.

## OBS. 81.

NOCTURNAL INCONTINENCE OF URINE; DUBIOUS RESULT.

A maid, aged 20 years. Orphaned a long time ago. Her father had always been a sickly man. She was brought up in an orphanage where many children peed in their beds. In the past she urinated in bed every night, more recently it only happens occasionally. However this problem has meant that she has to keep changing her employment. Since the 1 February 1891 when she started a new service, involuntary emission has occurred five times. The patient came to me under orders from her mistress on 15 March 1891. I treated her by hypnotic suggestion until the end of April 1891. During this period, the inconvenience only occurred once (the 21 March). I haven't seen her again nor had any further news of her.

## OBS. 82.

INCONTINENCE OF URINE AND FAECES DAY AND NIGHT. IMPROVEMENT.

An orphan girl aged 8 years, brought from a provincial orphanage and placed temporarily in an orphans' house in Amsterdam in order to allow her to follow my treatment. Timid and retiring, good health. Of her family history I only learnt that she had been maltreated by her step-mother; that cruel mother had, among other things, kicked her in the stomach. Neither the child nor the person who brought her to me, was able to say whether her problem dated from before or after that event.

Throughout the time that she has been at the orphanage, that is to say more than two years, she has involuntarily urinated and defecated both day and night. On examination of her abdomen and genitals I find no abnormality.

I treated the little girl from 10 October to 13 December 1891. She went into a deep sleep and I always had some difficulty in waking her.

In view of the gravity of the case, the results obtained during those two months could be described as satisfactory. The daytime incontinence was completely halted and the child learned to hold her urine for at least 3 or 4 hours.

|  |  |  |  |  |
|---|---|---|---|---|
| From 10 to 31 October | I counted 3 nights | | | |
| " | 1 to 30 November | " | " 11 | " |
| " | 1 to 13 December | " | " 9 | " |

that she remained free of her infirmity.

Notwithstanding this clear improvement, the head of the orphanage recalled the child without letting me know and without thanking me for my care (so grateful).

## OBS. 83.

INCONTINENCE OF URINE NIGHT AND DAY. FAILURE.

Young girl aged 13 years, excellent health and well constituted, periods haven't yet started.

The mother died of glycosuria, the father is neurasthenic. A younger brother pees in his bed. No internal or external lesions of abdominal or reproductive organs. No hysterical stigmata.

For four years the patient has been subject to involuntary emission of urine night and day. There are times however (rare it is true) that the problem disappears for several days. All the medicines have been tried. Hypnotic suggestion was applied by me for eleven months. I gave a session per day without obtaining the least improvement.

As well as direct suggestion I tried covert suggestion: suspension, faradisation.

## OBS. 84.

NOCTURNAL INCONTINENCE OF URINE, CHOREA, CURE.

A 12-year-old boy. Neurasthenic father. Subject to involuntary passing of urine once or twice a week, presenting the symptoms of unilateral chorea for several days. Bites his nails. Has been treated from 21 December 1892 until 31 January 1893. From the first session the incontinence disappeared. Complete cure of both infirmities, cure maintained, latest news dating from January 1894 leaves nothing to be desired.

## OBS. 85.

INCONTINENCE OF URINE DAY AND NIGHT. CURE.

Little girl, 8 years old, very agitated child, nervous but otherwise enjoying good health, complains of fleeting pains in the lower abdomen and irritation of the urethra. No lesions found in those areas. She can't hold on to her urine at a particular time, as soon as she feels the need to go to the toilet emission takes place. She passes urine 12 to 14 times a day, often without being aware of it. She pees in her bed every night.

Deep hypnosis. I treated this child from 26 August to 9 November 1889, with most satisfactory results. Her agitation calmed down, she succeeded in not feeling the need to urinate more than three or four times a day and the unconscious passage of urine disappeared completely both day and night. No relapse.

## OBS. 86.

NOCTURNAL INCONTINENCE OF URINE, MARKED IMPROVEMENT.

A 14-year-old boy, weak, debilitated, malnourished. Serious family history of nervous and psychological conditions. Is behind for his age, lazy, doesn't apply himself. No organic lesions. Irregular incontinence of urine. Sometimes a fortnight goes by without the appearance of any difficulty, then he pees in bed several days in a row.

Treated by hypnotic suggestion from September 1889 to July 1890.

Deep hypnosis. Improvement by all accounts. He is better nourished, has lost his bad moods and lazy habits, applies himself, only pees in his bed from time to time. As the parents were leaving town, the treatment was interrupted prematurely. No recent news.

## OBS. 87.

NOCTURNAL INCONTINENCE OF URINE, DECIDED IMPROVEMENT.

A 6-year-old boy of healthy parents pees in bed every night. Treated by hypnotic suggestion five times at great intervals from 12 October 1890 to 26 February 1890. Unconscious passage of urine only occurred rarely. No recent news.

## OBS. 88.

INCONTINENCE OF URINE, CURE.

A sweet little girl aged 10 years passes urine unconsciously every night. She is cured by suggestion in a state of deep sleep. Six sessions from 25 to 30 November 1889 were sufficient to achieve this result. Recurrence of problem after five weeks. One session of suggestion ended the cure which has been maintained ever since.

## OBS. 89.

INCONTINENCE OF URINE. FAILURE.

A young girl aged 18 years, of robust health. Involuntary passage of urine at night.

Family history of nervous trouble on the maternal side. Brought to consult me against her will. She is refractory to hypnotic manoeuvres. Suggestion in a waking state remains ineffective. Has abandoned the treatment.

## OBS. 90.

INCONTINENCE OF URINE DAY AND NIGHT, CURE.

For four years after recovering from scarlet fever, an 11-year-old girl has been subject to urinary incontinence both day and night. She pees up to three or four times an hour and feels incapable of holding her urine. She doesn't go to class for that reason. She is thin, bewildered, suffers from genital pruritus.

After one session of hypnotic suggestion, she recovered the ability to retain urine for two to three hours. After the third session the nocturnal incontinence was cured. Complete cure in a few days. Was treated from 20 January to 3 April 1890. No relapse.

## OBS. 91.

INCONTINENCE OF URINE DAY AND NIGHT. NOTABLE IMPROVEMENT.

A little boy aged 6 ½ years, wets his clothes at least once a day. At night he passes urine involuntarily sometimes two or three times. During the day he continually feels the need to pee, he often pees in his trousers without realising it.

After a first session of suggestion, he could hold his urine for at least an hour, after the second session he ceased to pee in his bed. At first I woke him up at night to pee, then I suggested that he get up spontaneously to satisfy his needs, a suggestion which he completely put into practice.

Was treated for three weeks. I haven't had news of him since then.

Out of a total 27 patients who were treated by hypnotic suggestion in our clinic between 15 August 1887 and 30 June 1893 we were able to record 14 cures, 1 dubious result, 6 enduring improvements, 3 transient improvements and 4 failures.

We also dare to suggest that this problem is among those which are particularly susceptible to cure by suggestion. Our results support those obtained by Messrs. Liébeault, Wetterstrand, Ringier and others.

In most cases treated by us the patients had been previously submitted to all sorts of different treatments, such as: being forced to lie on one side or on the stomach during sleep; inclination of the bed so that the head was lower than the feet; the application of leeches to the coccyx; mechanical compression of the urethra by an apparatus attached to the perineum, or even the agglutination of the prepuce by collodion; sitz baths and the washing of private parts with cold water; repeated awakening during the night, vermifuges, nux vomica, belladonna; electricity; and finally the operation of phimosis[87]. It was only as a last resort, and in desperation as to the cause that recourse to psycho-therapy occurred.

The majority of patients (21 out of 27) were aged 10 years or more, eight of them had attained or passed the age of puberty. Both sexes were represented in more or less equal numbers, we counted 13 boys and 14 girls.

In a third of cases, the patients had a family history of nerves or psychological disturbance.

---

[87] *Agglutination of the foreskin.

We often had to note relapses in patients who had been free of their problem for weeks or even months. Most often the relapses were precipitated by intercurrent illnesses or emotional states.

In the majority of cases we continued to observe the patients for a long time after the end of their treatment in order to confirm the duration and solidity of the cure.

Our treatment confines itself to provoking by verbal suggestion as deep a state of sleep as possible, and under those conditions suggesting to the patients that they will feel the need to pass urine during the night and will wake themselves and get up to urinate.

With those who don't achieve a deep sleep, we prolong the sessions for a gradually increasing amount of time, from 1 to 4 hours, in order to accustom patients to retain their urine throughout that period.

# A. GROUPE V.

## Neuralgias, Pains, Cramps.

It is particularly appropriate to reserve the domain of the neuralgias for the triumphs of the suggestive method. In the treatment of chronic cephalgia and of prosopalgia we have had great success. The majority of these cases demand a long lasting treatment and it is wise to prepare a patient for this before commencing his cure. It is absolutely essential that he takes on the idea that his illness is functional in nature and perfectly curable, but that he is vulnerable to relapses which are not to be feared when he knows that suggestion will cure him once again. In this way we avoid discouragement during a recurrence of pain. After the cure we continue to see our patients from time to time or even maintain contact by correspondence. In that way their moral support never falters, and we can be given due warning of an impending recurrence, which is then easier to cure than if the neuralgia is given time to anchor itself in the brain, thus a bit of salutary advice or a suggestion, given in time, can prevent a relapse.

Here again, it isn't the good sleepers who are mostly susceptible to cure, we have obtained some dazzling successes with patients who didn't get past the first degree of the hypnotic state.

## OBS. 92.

CHRONIC CEPHALGIA, CURE.

Towards the middle of June 1889 a lady aged 37 years, unmarried, asked me to treat her by suggestion for a recurrent headache.

After a stay of six weeks during which I gave her a session every day, the patient felt very relieved but wasn't completely cured. Circumstances forced her to interrupt the treatment but she promised to come back to see me as soon as she could. In fact, on the following 1 October she resumed treatment and I had the satisfaction of curing her. From the 15 November she was able to leave me, completely rid of her headache.

Miss T. had lost her parents at a young age and was taken in by an aunt. As far as she knew there was no family history of nervous disease.

After her cure, my ex-patient continued to give me news from time to time. In October 1893, thus four years afterwards, she was kind enough to send me the following account of her illness and the cure which I had given her:

Dear Doctor,

I can ask no more than to give you an account of my illness and the cure which you carried out.

You understand better than anybody what pleasure it gives me to enlarge upon my cure by suggestive treatment.

From my earliest youth I suffered from headaches. I often had to miss school because of my cephalgia. As I got older the headaches gradually got worse in intensity and frequency. I was medicated in vain. I spent terrible nights, full of dreams, and I always woke up with a painful heavy head. Sometimes the pain diminished during the course of the day, but most often it persisted and sometimes there were periods of two to three weeks when I was continually disturbed my my headache.

Every morning on getting up I had nausea and vomiting. I felt unable to eat. The sickness accompanied by a feeling of weakness stayed with me all morning.

I felt more and more nervous, prickly, irritated by the slightest thing. That mental state led to a disgust with life, a total depression of my being. I often spent hours crying in a corner when I thought no one could see me.

I felt unable to combat this sadness which obsessed me. I couldn't understand how I had ever been able to study and take the examinations for my teaching diploma. I tried everything I could think of to get rid of my headaches but nothing worked. So when suggestion and hypnotism was recommended, it was only reluctantly and without the least hope of a cure that I decided to consult you.

No doubt you remember my restlessness during the early days, I wasn't able to sleep, your suggestions didn't have the least effect on me! It's only thanks to your inexhaustible patience and your immovable conviction that gradually your words made an impression on me, that your suggestions were realised, that an ineffable calm came over me during the session, and that I was filled with faith in psycho-therapy.

Gradually the cure manifested itself, I had better nights, my head felt liberated in the mornings, intermittent headaches replaced the permanent pain, the bouts diminished in strength and frequency. As a result my general state also changed. Whereas I had been morose and taciturn I became cheerful and lighthearted.

It's four years now since I was cured, I still remember perfectly each suggestion that you made to me, your words seem to be anchored in my brain, they support me, strengthen my courage, they continue to keep me on the right path.

All your predictions were realised. I no longer have that terrible headache. Nobody who hasn't suffered from headaches can possibly understand what it feels like to be rid of them.

I tell you frankly that I only learnt to enjoy and appreciate life after my cure etc. etc.

## OBS. 93.

CHRONIC CEPHALGIA. CURE.

Mr S., an engineer, aged 54 years, having passed most of his life in the Indies, was referred to me by a colleague in order to rid him of a tenacious headache refractory to treatment with drugs.

The patient is a robust man who doesn't seem his age. He suffered a lot from cephalgia whilst in the colonies. The beginning of the headaches dates from a journey he made from Batavia to Saigon and was precipitated by a chill. He did his best to cure himself but nothing worked. The aches are not regular but are triggered by sudden changes in temperature and by emotions. They always begin in the forehead above his eyes, mainly the left eye, radiate from there to the top of his head and thence to the occipital area or towards the mastoid apophysis or they localise in a scar from a wound caused by a fragment of stone. These pains sometimes persist for a whole series of days, sometimes they disappear after a few hours.

In April 1890 after having been ill with influenza, Mr Sch. was troubled by his cephalgia regularly every day. The bout of headaches would start at about 4.30pm and wouldn't go away until 10 o'clock at night. The pain was resistant to all treatment.

In all other ways his health left nothing to be desired. The patient is a nervy man very easily driven to anger. From time to time he feels giddy. No heart trouble, no arteriosclerosis.

On the 23 July 1890 at 11 o'clock in the morning, thus at a time when the patient wasn't suffering from his neuralgia, I put him to sleep. My suggestion, notably that the headache would not occur after dinner, was perfectly realised. After a second session the neuralgia which had happened regularly every day for months, disappeared for good.

However the hypnosis that I obtained scarcely went further than the state of somnolence.

I saw the patient again from time to time afterwards in order to consolidate the cure which was maintained.

Mr. Sch. spent the following year in Java once again. He remained free of his headaches.

## OBS. 94.

SPASMODIC FUNCTIONAL CONTRACTURE OF THE HANDS. CURE.

A small rentier, retired for some time from a potato business, came to consult me and asked to be cured of a contracture of both his hands. The patient is a man of athletic build, seems healthy and nothing less than nervous. He is 75 years old. His right hand is altogether closed, the four fingers are contracted inwards forming a fist, only his thumb remains unaffected and can move freely. There is atrophy of the interosseous muscles. The left hand is unaffected save for the ring and middle fingers. These two fingers also show the beginnings of an inward contracture. The patient thinks that the right hand began to become deformed about ten years ago. He attributes his problem to his profession as a seller which involved measuring out potatoes all the time, which required repeated flexion of his hand.

*Family history.*

At the age of 20 years, after having looked after a mentally ill uncle for some time, the patient contracted a nervous state that persisted for a few days, giving rise to insomnia and general torpor. He was cured by narcotic medication. He is subject to nervous tremors which date from that time. They occur when he intends to carry out a small movement, for example moving a queen in a game of draughts. He became very nervous at one time due to overwork whilst learning German. He comes from a family of neuropaths.

A trial of opening the fingers of his right hand didn't succeed and caused him pain.

Although I had little hope of curing the patient with suggestion, I thought that his family and personal history of nerves warranted a try. Against expectation the patient proved to be very suggestible. I was able to induce a state of deep sleep and several sessions of suggestion even allowed me to passively open his hand, then to have the hand open actively without pain. I got the patient to carry out methodical exercises with his fingers and I had the satisfaction of completely conquering the contraction over a period of about three months.

## OBS. 95.

SACRO-LUMBAR NEURALGIA, CURE BY SUGGESTION IN THE WAKING STATE IN A SINGLE SESSION.

A teacher at a lycée, married for three months, suffering since his marriage from neuralgic pains in the left sacro-lumbar region. He is 32 years old, is unaware of any personal or family history of nerves, was addicted to masturbation from the age of 13 to 15 years, never cohabited before his marriage.

There is a clear relation between the exacerbation of his neuralgia and his sexual relations. Although he has spontaneously reduced his sexual activity, and even though those relations have not occurred more than once a week for some time, he has noticed that the second or third day or more after coitus a serious bout of neuralgia occurs. Very worried by this nervous condition which imposes frequent absences from his lessons and hasn't got any better after treatment instituted by his regular doctor, he asked me to give him my opinion.

A thorough examination of the affected region and the genitals of the patient confirmed the absolute absence of all organic pathology.

I reassured the patient with authority that from that moment he would be able to have sexual relations with his wife without any fear and without the act giving rise to a recurrence of his neuralgia. That suggestion given in a decisive tone had an excellent effect.

Indeed from then on the pains stopped happening. The cure has not been refuted for four years.

## OBS. 96.

CHRONIC SCIATICA DATING BACK SIX YEARS, CURE.

On the 2 September 1890, a married man aged 38 years suffering from a congenital subluxation of the right hip, came to consult me for neuralgic pains located in the whole of his right lower limb.

These pains appeared for the first time in his hip and right buttock after a chill. He has had them now for six years.

He first noticed them on the night following a forced three hour march. All sweaty and tired out, he had sat down on a stone bench to have a rest. Since then the pains haven't left him, however he has noticed some intermittent periods of relief, of variable duration but never longer than five or six days. The pains are normally quite bearable, but occasionally very painful attacks occur. The patient has undergone various treatments: he has been treated with blistering poultices, massage, and electricity without gaining any serious benefit. Easily hypnotisable, he goes to sleep deeply as soon as I close his eyes. On waking all the pain has disappeared. Treatment by hypnotic suggestion, repeated every day for a week then at gradually increasing intervals, was continued until the following 5 December. The pains didn't reappear during the whole of that time. No further news received.

## OBS. 97.

CHRONIC SCIATICA FOR SIX YEARS, HYSTERICAL SYMPTOMS, CURE.

A married lady aged 47 years, came to consult me on the 1 August 1891 asking me to cure her of a sciatica which had been troubling her for about six years. She was born in the Dutch-Indies from an indigenous mother and a Dutch father. She lost her parents at a very young age. She married a neurasthenic man at the age of 36 and has one child from that marriage, a little girl aged 7 years who is excessively nervous. The patient often has headaches, a lump in her throat and hyperaesthesiae of the scalp. In July 1873, during a season she spent at Wiesbade, she had an attack of *alopecia areata*[88] for the first time. Five or six perfectly bald circular patches developed on the top of her head. After about a year some silky hair grew back and soon fell out to be replaced definitively by normal hair. The patches of alopecia were painful.

The sciatica began in 1885 without any obvious cause. The neuralgic pains had prolonged periods of noticeable improvement and serious exacerbations condemning the patient to complete rest, however she has never ceased to be troubled by them.

Last January, reappearance of alopecia. There are now two round bald patches on the top of her head which are very painful.

On examination of her leg I find no painful points and no signs of muscular atrophy. Movement is painful and tiring. The patient suffers a great deal, mainly at night when she shifts her position. She avoids going out of her home as much as possible, not only because walking is painful but also because of the pain she gets in her head when she is wearing her hat.

Easy hypnosis. Light sleep. Great suggestibility. After a quarter of an hour's sleep the patient wakes up free of her pains.

At intervals of two or three days, I continue my hypnotic suggestions for six weeks. The pains reappear at the beginning of treatment after a variable amount of time, be it spontaneously, be it after an emotion, from tiredness or a sudden change in temperature.

---

[88] * Patchy hair loss.

From the second half of the cure they disappear for good. No relapse, even after six months.

## OBS. 98.

TIC DOULEREUX DATING BACK 25 YEARS. VERY DECIDED IMPROVEMENT.

Mrs A. B. of a healthy but delicate constitution is a nervous frail person. She is 50 years old, is married and has suffered from tic douloureux since her 25th year, with free intervals lasting from several days to six or seven months.

Changes in atmospheric conditions, emotions, and intercurrent illnesses are the most frequent triggers for a recurrence of her pains. At different times the patient has undergone appropriate treatments, she has tried many and consulted the most renowned specialists and authorities, without achieving a permanent cure.

On the 29 September 1888, Mrs A. B. having been suffering from her spasmodic, painful tic on the right side of her face for several weeks, came to see me for the first time at the insistence of her doctor.

She sleeps little, eats badly, speaks in a low voice, avoids all movement of her head which isn't absolutely necessary. The exacerbations of pain usually occur in the mornings after getting dressed. Apart from these neuralgic symptoms the patient complains of heart palpitations and congestive pressure in her neck and face. She believes she is at risk of apoplexy. She is very irritable and cries for no reason.

No hysterical stigmata, nothing abnormal regarding her heart. Serious family history of nervous conditions.

I give a hypnotic suggestive session on four consecutive days. Light hypnosis, satisfactory suggestibility. The pains, the spasmodic tic, the palpitations, disappear and come back sometime after the sessions. The nights are better, her general state improves, the hope of a cure is reborn. The patient asks me to give her a break of several days to sort out her affairs promising to come back to see me as soon as possible.

I saw the patient again on the 10 of the following December. Her condition was very much improved, so much so that she at first thought she was cured. She remained in treatment until the 18 January 1889.

The hypnotic sleep that I obtain is very deep. After a few sessions all the nervous symptoms disappeared; from then on I distanced my suggestions more and more. On the day of her departure, Mrs A. B. hadn't felt any neuralgia for three weeks.

It was only at the end of March 1890, thus fourteen months later, that the patient came again for a minor relapse. A marriage planned for her only daughter had made her emotional and set off the tic and the pain. Fifteen days sufficed perfectly to reestablish the normal state of affairs. The hypnosis induced was much deeper this time than last year. Since then I haven't had any further news.

The following observation is interesting in more than one regard. First it teaches us once more that neurectomy is no guarantee against relapses. In fact we know that a lasting cure obtained by this operative procedure has only been noted in about 3% of cases[89]. Secondly the very special effect that aconitine produced in the patient, gives food for thought. Is there reason to think that the elective action of that alkaloid on the trigeminal nerve, manifesting itself in sensations of engorgement and prickliness in the regions served by that nerve, produce a suggestive action on the patient, leading in certain appropriate cases, to a cure? We are inclined to believe it. In the final analysis it comes down to this observation: that suggestion cleverly masked can cure a tenacious and resistant neuralgia, where simple suggestion has failed. Quite simply it's a question of making use of the same process by finding a weak point in the armour. When a relapse occurred and the patient didn't even seek my care, a consultation with a somnambulist and his prescriptions had a salutary effect on his imagination.

Also when the patient did come to see me a long time afterwards, I had no reason to undermine his faith in the effect obtained and I advised him to resume that treatment if the pains should ever come back.

---

[89] Comp.: Jurgensen, Lehrbuch der Suez., Pathos. und Therap. S. 9. 1886.

## OBS. 99.

TIC DOULOUREUX DATING BACK THREE YEARS. NEURECTOMY. PERSISTENCE OF NEURALGIA. CURE BY SUGGESTION. RELAPSE. NEW CURE.

Mr W. aged 49 years, a businessman in a large market town some distance away, was referred to me by his doctor on 24 March 1891.

The patient had already been suffering from a neuralgia of the second and third branches of the right trigeminal nerve for three years. Electricity, medicine and as a last resort neurectomy were the mainstays of a very thorough treatment on the part of my colleague.

When a recurrence of pain occurred a fortnight after the excision of part of the nerve and injection of high doses of morphine didn't succeed in alleviating it, he asked me to try psycho-therapy.

The patient is a man of medium height, without any family history of nervous complaints. He had never had any serious illnesses nor suffered from any nervous problems before he was affected by prosopalgia. For almost three years the pains have given him little respite. As he has tried nearly all the recommended treatments without obtaining any serious benefit, he has become very sceptical and only submitted to my procedures on the insistence of his doctor.

He is melancholic, has bad nights, lacks appetite, is very thin. A very irritable man, he avoids movement as much as possible, he scarcely dares to open his mouth.

The acts of speaking, chewing and swallowing, trigger or exacerbate the pain. During his multiple crises, tears, nasal mucus and saliva wet his face and at the same time a convulsive tic makes him grimace. A grinding of teeth and guttural noises often accompany these symptoms.

While the friend who accompanied the patient was describing his case, Mr W. had an attack of pain.

I succeeded in calming him by verbal suggestion and by light passes, a calm that I was able to maintain for an hour, however the patient did not sleep. I saw the patient again every day at the same time. My suggestions had the effect of bringing an improvement in his condition in so far as he slept better at night and the pains diminished in intensity.

On the 31 March the patient didn't come at the usual time, he was late by nearly an hour and excused himself saying that a terrible fit of neuralgia had delayed him. He hadn't been able to resist the temptation and had given himself an injection of 65 mg. of morphine. Profiting from the sedation which came over him afterwards he brought himself to my session.

The session was no different to previous ones. The effect of the morphine injection, the momentary sedation, didn't noticeably increase the effect of my suggestions.

On the 2 April an attack of pain occurred during the hypnotic state.

Despairing of achieving my goal by suggestion alone, I decided to call upon the known action of aconitine as an anti-neuralgic. I maintained the daily sessions of suggestion while at the same time prescribing crystalline granules of aconitine in doses of ⅛ mg. to be taken as 1 granule every hour to a maximum of 4 granules.

The patient was to take the first granule in the evenings at 6 o'clock, the last at 9 o'clock.

The next day in his session, he told me that he had a good night and described the effect the granules had like a sensation of painful heaviness coming from his brain and radiating towards the periphery whereas the usual pain during an attack was felt first in his face and moved from there towards his head. He preferred the aconitine's centrifugal sensation to the centripetal pain of the tic. When the action of the aconitine was exhausted, the painful heaviness was followed by a reparative sleep.

*7 May.* The mixed treatment has been continued. There hasn't been a single attack of tic properly so called. However the patient continues to speak in a low voice and avoids chewing, feeding himself with soups, raw eggs and milk. He lives in constant fear of a recurrence of the tic which exacerbates his pain.

From today I stop the aconitine and forcefully reason with him. I give him to understand that there is no longer any question of an organic lesion, or a neurological condition properly so called, and that his pains are psychological in nature deriving from his imagination which is always active, the excision of part of the nerve having paralysed the peripheral source of pain and the action of the aconitine having relieved the central nervous system. I urge him to force himself to speak in a loud voice, to share the family meals, to eat all the dishes, to rinse his mouth in the morning and clean his teeth, to wash in cold water etc etc in brief: to act as if he no longer had any pain and as if he no longer feared having any pain. After this little speech I succeeded for the first time in putting the patient to sleep. In fact a light sleep.

*8 May.* Yesterday's session had an excellent effect. The patient took a stroll for two hours and didn't stop talking to himself in a loud voice throughout that time. He took his meals with the family and ate everything without having any pain. From today he will add two litres of milk to his regular diet.

*12 May.* The patient is over the moon, he feels completely rid of his tic. I allow him to go home and come and see me once a week, as long as he follows my advice to the letter. The cure lasts until the following 5 October. A minor relapse triggered by the cold, followed by relief after a few days.

On the following 20 October the patient left me for good, he couldn't spend any more time away from his business, especially in the winter. I recommended him to give himself a session of suggestion at home every day at the same time. I gave him the appropriate suggestions in writing that he was to read before going to sleep.

From time to time the patient provided me with his news which was excellent, however from February 1892 I heard nothing more.

Two months later I learnt he had been sick with influenza following which a serious recurrence of his tic had occurred.

For very good reasons it was impossible for him to come to Amsterdam to have the care I was offering him.

On the 5 of the following September Mr W. paid me a visit, perfectly radiant and free of his tic. On asking him if the pains had disappeared spontaneously he confessed that no, he had suffered a lot and it wasn't until after he had undertaken treatment recommended by a somnambulist living in a nearby town, whom he consulted at the instigation of a friend, that the cure had been effected. The treatment was composed of a winey extract of various herbs prescribed by the oracle, of which he had to drink three little glasses per day, and some magnetic passes that his wife had to make over him every day at the same time. The cure had taken a month, but from that time onwards he had been delivered from his pain.

I congratulated him on the success obtained and I strongly advised him not to depart from the advice that the somnambulist had given him, at the same time asking him to continue to keep me informed of his progress from time to time.

The latest news dates from February 1894. He has experienced a short-lived relapse two or three times at intervals of several months, but every time the resumption of the treatment prescribed by the somnambulist has been effective in making the pain disappear.

## OBS. 100.

RIGHT PROSOPALGIA, CURE IN THREE SUGGESTIVE SESSIONS.

Mrs Z. aged 40 years, is married but has no children. For several years she has suffered from neuralgia of the third branch of the right trigeminal nerve. Her dentist has extracted all her affected teeth. She is left with no more than two molars in good condition. Rather than extract these last two teeth, the dentist advises the patient to come and consult me.

5 January 1893. No hysterical stigmata, no family history of nervous conditions. The tic occurs at intervals of several months and continues, notwithstanding the fact that the decayed tooth which originally triggered the pain was removed. She often suffers from her neuralgia for weeks on end. She has been ill now for a fortnight. She replies to my questions, mouth closed and clenching her teeth, she dares not even swallow her saliva for fear of triggering an attack.

Saying some calming words to her I proceed with the occlusion of her eyes. Calm is immediately established, her respiration slows, her tears cease to flow, the patient goes to sleep. I suggest the disappearance of her pain and after a few minutes I wake her up. I saw the patient again on the day after next. She had continued to be pain free until that morning. On waking she felt a little pain behind her ear and fearing a relapse she had come to ask me to put her to sleep and to suggest the complete disappearance of her pain, which I did. After the session there were no further complaints.

I heard news of this patient from her dentist on 5 November 1893. The tic had not recurred.

## OBS. 101.

TIC DOULEREUX DATING BACK ONE YEAR, CURE BY HYPNOTIC SUGGESTION.

Mr K. is a nervous irascible man. He retired from business two years ago and lives with his wife off rents. He is 60 years old, has no children. No individual or family history of nervous complaints.

His neuralgia dates from July 1891. At first his right cheek became very sensitive. Cold water bothered him, contact with it made him feel as if his jaw was dislocated. The hyperaesthesia gave way to a dull pain, to intermittent sharp stabbing pains and finally to attacks of neuralgia. The pains started from behind his ear and radiated along his cheek towards his nose, ear and right side of his chin. The doctor diagnosed a tic douloureux but his treatment scarcely provided any relief for the patient. Mr K. consulted different doctors in turn and tried out various treatments, most recently he was treated by electricity. His pain disappeared during the sessions, only to come back afterwards. He had all his teeth extracted on the affected side. A morphine injection given during an attack made him so ill that he preferred the pain to the side effects of the remedy.

*Present state* 27 September 1892.

Mr K. is accompanied by his wife who describes her husband's case to me. He seems fine for his 60 years, he is sitting with his head bent, resting on his right hand, tears overflowing on his face, from time to time he grinds his teeth and moans. The attacks happen at intervals varying between a few minutes to two hours. He sleeps little and rarely more than two hours at a time. He eats irregularly in the intervals between attacks. Draughts, emotions, the act of speaking, coughing, sneezing, chewing, swallowing, set off the pain.

Nothing relieves him during an attack with the exception of a hot cataplasm. The pain starts sometimes in the mastoid hypophysis spreading towards his cheek, his tongue and his chin, sometimes it starts in his lower jaw and radiates toward his eye and right ear.

The patient is very suggestible. I succeed in putting him to sleep at the first attempt and in ridding him of his pains. From 27 September to 10 October I give one session of hypnotic suggestion every day then one every two days until 21 October. All the symptoms disappear and the patient believes himself cured. However on 21 October Mr K. following a fit of anger had a recurrence of his tic. Another session put paid to his pain. I continued the treatment gradually spacing out the sessions until the 2 December. On that date I declared him cured.

During the course of the year 1893 he came to consult me twice, notably in March and at the end of October for a minor recurrence.

A few sessions sufficed to assure a cure on both occasions.

## OBS. 102.

CHRONIC CEPHALGIA AND SPASMODIC TIC, NOTABLE IMPROVEMENT.

A young 16-year-old girl, good constitution, strong for her age and seeming to be in excellent health, menarche two years ago, referred to me by a colleague.

She has been affected for some time by a spasmodic tic of the frontal and pyramidal muscles of the nose and the elevators of the nostril and upper lip. The tremor and contractions occur in the form of attacks following the experience of certain emotions, or even if she just thinks about them, or her attention is directed toward them. She also complains of bouts of headaches occurring intermittently. Sometimes the headache lasts for three or four weeks, other times it only makes a fleeting appearance.

Other than this, her health leaves nothing to be desired. There is no family history of nervous complaints, no hysterical stigmata.

I treated this patient from 27 September 1892 to 17 February 1893. She was very suggestible and easily fell into a deep sleep. The headache was the first to cede to my suggestions and no longer occurred from the second half of October. The spasmodic tic gradually reduced in intensity and frequency, also from 4 November I was able to space out the sessions more and more.

During December and January the patient's state was so much improved that I only saw her from one fortnight to another. I gave her a last session on 17 February. She assured me that she hadn't been disturbed by her tic for at least three weeks, the headache had disappeared completely.

I told the patient to come back and see me if ever the symptoms threatened to reappear. I haven't heard news of her since.

## OBS. 103.

GASTRO-INTESTINAL NEURALGIA. UNILATERAL OVARIECTOMY. PERSISTANCE OF THE NEURALGIA. DECIDED IMPROVEMENT AS A RESULT OF PSYCHO-THERAPY.

Miss L. has been suffering from almost continual pains in her abdomen for several years. She underwent an oophorectomy in 1890 without benefitting in any way from that operation.

The pains are vague, not well localised, never go away completely and from time to time present exacerbations of a colicky type. The worst pains occur mainly in the region of her stomach. Her appetite is good, digestion is fine and there is no heartburn. Bowel movements are retarded. Tiredness aggravates the pain. The patient is assistant to a pharmacist and finds herself unable to do her job because standing up tires her too much. No hysterical stigmata, no other morbid symptoms.

Miss L. has been treated by different doctors, she has followed various treatments, has been operated on and underwent a Mitchel-Playfair cure without obtaining any relief.

On examination I note a slight heightening and an exaggerated sensitivity in the stomach region. The abdominal walls are thin and flaccid. Absence of the right ovary. There are no circumscribed, localised pains.

Subjected to the hypnotic procedures the patient reached the state of charm. She never went further than this first degree of influence. However hypnosis calmed her and diminished her pains. She was treated from 10 September 1891 to 21 of the following November. She left me very much improved, feeling able to resume her occupation serving in a pharmacy.

Some time afterwards I had a visit from Miss L. who continued to be well. She promised to come back to me if ever a recurrence of her pain occurred.

## OBS. 104.

GASTRALGIA LINKED IN ALL PROBABILITY TO A SCARRED STOMACH ULCER, CURE

Mrs P. A. aged 40 years suffered from gastralgia between the ages of 14 and 18. At the age of 18, following a gynaecological treatment, the pain disappeared. At the age of 25 a recurrence of the gastralgia and a cure after the same treatment. However, some time afterwards there was another recurrence, and since then her gastralgia has been resistant to all treatment. On one occasion a massive haematemesis occurred. The patient no longer remembers exactly when.

The pain is located in the epigastrium and radiates from there towards the two ovaries. The pain is most often accompanied by distension of the abdomen. The disappearance of the gastralgia and the pseudotympanites is not accompanied by eructations.

No appetite. Solid food causes pain. Pains occur randomly, sometimes they last for several hours on end, they are so bad that the patient cries out loud and and has to lie down and rest. During the last fortnight before she started my treatment, she suffered from gastralgia every day.

The patient is thin and looks debilitated and anaemic. Internal organs, including genital organs (with the exception of her stomach), show no anatomical abnormality. No ovaralgia, no meteorism[90], no serious displacement of the stomach. There is a circumscribed pain under the xiphoid process of the sternum. The area is tender under pressure. When an attack occurs, her face becomes pale, the patient groans with pain, undoes her corset and lies down. No hysterical stigmata. Mrs P. A. has never had any other neuralgias. In recent times she has fed herself on eggs and milk that she finds easy to digest. She doesn't vomit and has no other dyspeptic symptoms. In the past she often vomited.

Ephemeral hypnosis. There isn't a sleepy sensation. However during the session the patient is completely relaxed and realises my

---

[90] * Abdominal distension.

suggestion admirably. Hypnotised during a gastralgic attack, the pain gave way to suggestion after a few moments. When the session continued a little longer the pain reappeared, however it consistently went away again after the simple application of my hand on her epigastrium.

The patient began her treatment of the 17 November 1889. The morbid condition improved immediately. After a fortnight the pains only appeared exceptionally and the patient tolerated and digested solid food perfectly well.

Since then she has only been treated intermittently at great intervals, notably on days when she has the pains. The cure was obtained after about three months . A relapse occurred in 1891 and was followed by a cure after a few days treatment.

At the present time (December 1893), the cure has not been refuted.

## OBS. 105.

MULTIPLE CHRONIC NEURALGIAS IN A HYSTERIC, REFRACTORY TO VARIOUS TREATMENTS, CURED BY HYPNOTIC SUGGESTION.

Miss A.v.T. aged 40 years, was born to nervous parents. She lost her mother at a very young age. Her father is still alive. Although he is nervous, he is a robust old man in excellent health. A younger sister had petit-mal fits and bouts of catalepsy before her marriage, since then her state has degenerated into fits of epilepsy. One of the patient's brothers presents the phenomenon of hyperhidrosis[91] from time to time localised to half of his face.

Miss V. T. enjoyed good health before her 18th year. Her illness dates from that time. One evening, being with friends in the country, she unwisely stayed outside too long on a balcony. The cold night air caught her and she became seriously chilled.

On the next day she had her first bout of enteralgia which was resistant to the treatment instituted for a long time.

Since then the domain of the neuralgia has successively extended, at first to contiguous regions, then to other areas more or less far away from the original site. The pains are felt sometimes in her abdomen, sometimes in the gastric region, on the front of her thorax, in her breast, in her back. They have a neuralgic character and are often accompanied by digestive troubles: reflux, acidity, nausea and vomiting, feelings of heaviness, loss of or capricious appetite, bradypepsia[92], constipation, diarrhoea, pseudo-tympanites and hysterical globus.

At irregular intervals the patient suffers from atrocious migraine. The hemicrania usually affects the left side of her face. The left eye has been affected by a detached retina fro some years. Serious myopia in both eyes. Sometimes the patient feels pain in her left ear.

This condition has existed since the year 1889 with periods of improvement and exacerbation. The different phenomena occur

---

[91] * Excessive sweating.

[92] * Slow digestion.

alternately in isolation or together, they are often accompanied by insomnia and giddiness, rarely by momentary loss of consciousness, never by epileptiform fits.

She has been treated by various doctors without obtaining any longterm benefit.

On the 14 November 1891 she placed herself under my care. A thorough examination having been undertaken which only revealed a functional disorder, I assured the patient that my treatment would in all probability cure her as long as she followed the regime I was going to prescribe in every detail and promised to abstain from all medication, whatever it might be, from now on.

Miss v. T. kept her promise, she never allowed herself the least deviation from the prescribed regime. The treatment was pursued until the 17 June 1892. I gave her daily sessions lasting about an hour. Light hypnosis, satisfactory suggestibility. The hypnosis always provided her with a state of agreeable calmness, her symptoms most often ceded to my suggestions. If they occasionally grew refractory or were slow to disappear I extended the sessions for two or three hours.

Miss v. T.'s general state was so much improved by June 1892 that she was able to allow herself a trip abroad for several weeks. After that, I saw her again from time to time at longer intervals in order to consolidate the treatment.

In January 1893 a serious relapse of enteralgia and nervous dyspepsia occurred. From 30 January to 26 February I submitted her to a special dietary cure at the same time as giving her extended suggestive hypnotic sessions every day. This treatment was followed by a cure which has so far not been challenged. The latest news dates from September 1894.

A lady L. asked me if I would look after her child suffering from prolapse of the of the anus, which reminded me of an analogous case I had seen treated and cured by Doctor Liébault using suggestion. So I made a trial, which was moreover, crowned with success.

**OBS. 106.**

ANAL PROLAPSE IN A 5-YEAR-OLD CHILD, CURE BY HYPNOTIC SUGGESTION.

Mrs L. who had been cured of hysterical melancholia and chronic constipation by hypnotic suggestion (See Obs. 58) told me one day about one of her children, a lively little boy and otherwise very healthy, affected by anal prolapse. The doctors she had consulted shrugged their shoulders telling her that it would pass. Wishing to see her child rid of this embarrassing and painful trouble she asked me to kindly take on her son. The problem had already been going on for two years, after the least effort the intestine came out and would often only go back in hours later after the application of warm towels. On the mother's insistence I agreed to see her child.

I asked the mother to sit down in an armchair and hold her son on her knees. Then I proceeded to put both the mother and child to sleep without any difficulty. Then I applied my hand for some time to the little patient's tummy suggesting to him all the while in a soft voice that he was no longer the little boy he had been in the past, that he would go to the toilet once or twice every day without needing to make any serious effort and that his intestine would no longer come out. After six sessions (each of about half an hour) given at intervals of two or three days, the cure was obtained. Eighteen months have now passed since the effect was obtained without any relapse having occurred.

## B. GROUPS VI and VII.
## Illnesses of diverse organs or systems,
(OTHER THAN THE NERVOUS SYSTEM).

It is easy to foresee, now that nearly everybody agrees on the preponderant role that suggestion plays in all treatments, now that the immense influence of the psychological over the physical is recognised by everyone, that psycho-therapy will not be neglected in illnesses or so called organic accidents, be they external or internal, and will be indicated as a complement to all other treatments.

We repeat together with Bernheim: " One can only cure what is curable; one can relieve and often improve what is incurable."

There is a nervous element very much in every illness, functional disorders are easily superimposed on organic disorder. Often, very often, the doctor — even the most gifted — fails to detect it, makes a mistaken diagnosis. In many cases, if he knows how to use suggestion, it will help him to recognise the problem.

In the various cases confided to our care, we have been able to shorten and slightly diminish the frequency of true cardiac angina attacks, thus allowing the poor patients to get some sleep at night, we weren't able to prevent a recurrence of their attacks; for arthritics and rheumatics, suggestion has been able to mitigate their pain thus allowing them to reduce their medication to a minimum. Attacks of asthma symptomatic of an organic heart lesion seemed to us less difficult for the patients to bear under the influence of suggestion.

Suggestion addressing itself to functional problems can — in so far as the organic state allows it — ameliorate the symptoms and in thus restoring function contribute to the organic recovery.

## B. GROUP VIII.
## Anaemia. Menstrual abnormalities.

We have only dealt with a very limited number of cases in this category. It isn't that we failed in the case of anaemias nor that menstrual abnormalities haven't been treated by us. It's rather that the people affected by these disorders have also required our care for other concurrent morbid states.

In the rare case where anaemia or menstrual irregularity alone were the object of treatment, the effect obtained was of the best.

The anaemics proved to be easily hypnotisable and very suggestible.

## C. GROUP IX.

### Surgical anaesthesia.

Hypnotism can render excellent service as a means of preventing pain in surgical operations and during childbirth. In some subjects it can replace chloroform. However hypnotic analgesia will never dethrone anaesthesia with chloroform. In recent publications and in French and German reviews of hypnotism, different authors have reported cases of surgical anaesthesia. We refer to the publications of Messrs. Dumontpallier, Mesnet, Delboeuf, Wetterstrand, Bourdon, von Schrenck-Notzing, Tatzel, Schmeltz and others. For ourselves we have to note some successes suggesting we should not neglect the power of suggestion in appropriate cases.

### OBS. 107.

COMPLETE RUPTURE OF THE PERINEUM DATING BACK SEVERAL YEARS. RADICAL OPERATION WITHOUT NOTABLE PAIN, UNDER THE INFLUENCE OF SUGGESTION WITHOUT SLEEP[93]

On the 7th March 1892, Mr.N. accompanied by his wife, came to consult me. Mrs N. is 34 years old and apparently enjoys excellent

---

[93] See: Revue de l'hypnotisme. Janvier 1893.
Zeitschrift für Hypnotismus. 1893. Heft IV.

health, she is slightly inclined towards obesity. She is the mother of four children. Since her last confinement, dating back several years already, she has been very troubled by a complete tear of the perineum.

Doctor Mr. de L., gynaecologist, when consulted about it, advised her to undergo a radical but painful operation.

Mrs N., knowing herself to be very sensitive to pain, objects that since the operation is so painful she could not submit herself to it, seeing that the doctor who looked after her in the past for a heart condition said that a narcotisation with chloroform could be fatal.

An examination carried out confirmed an organic condition of the heart in compensation. And so I had to respond to a question put by her husband in the affirmative: " Could chloroformisation in this case expose the patient to deadly risks?" Mr N. then enquired whether there were not other procedures for obtaining analgesia. We discussed an anaesthetic method advocated by a German doctor, to the effect that: multiple hypodermic injections of minimal doses of a very weak solution of cocaine are given throughout the operation as and when necessary. The analgesia obtained in that way would exclude all risks and allow major operations to be carried out without pain, for example mastectomies. Cocaine was just as frightening as chloroform. In the end we discussed local anaesthesia by freezing and it was agreed that it could only be used in order to allow the initial skin incision to be made painlessly. They were going to abandon the whole idea of an operation when Dr M. de L., recalling some surgical anaesthesia obtained by suggestion, suggested Mr and Mrs N. come to ask my advice.

In this case, the suggestive method being the last resort, I opined bravely to the patient that hypnotism would work for her. So I asked the lady to come to see me every day at the same time assuring her that my repeated suggestions would not take long to produce the desired anaesthesia.

As much as she feared the pain, Mrs N. also wanted to be rid of her problem. Also her assiduousness in being hypnotised was exemplary. However in spite of her good will, sleep didn't happen. I was only able to achieve a light feeling of beatitude for my patient, only a state of more or less somnolence. Predicting that this state of affairs would alarm her, I took care from the beginning to suggest to her that sleep, properly so called, wasn't absolutely necessary, and that a state of somnolence would suffice for the realisation of my suggestions of analgesia. I backed up my assertion by giving her needle pricks on her arm during the session, pricks that she imagined hurting much less than when she was completely awake. Then I stimulated her imagination by extracting a tooth from a lady who was awake without causing any pain. That lady had been put to sleep many times by me and was very suggestible.

I appealed to her *amour-propre,* I repeated over and again that her wish to vanquish the pain and not to feel it was growing with every session. I promised to be present at the operation, that I would continue my suggestions throughout its duration, finally I assured her that I was perfectly convinced she would acquit herself wonderfully and would scarcely suffer.

So I informed my colleague, Dr M. de L., of the readiness of his patient and he fixed the date of the operation for the following 24 April. On the 21 of that month Mrs N. went into the gynaecological clinic where I continued to give her a session every evening. The night of the 23/24 April was excellent. Mrs N. had a good sleep, she gave little signs of agitation when I saw her the moment before she was admitted into the operating theatre.

The operation began at about ten o'clock and was finished at quarter to eleven.

The first skin incision was preceded by local anaesthesia with *ethyl chloride,* after that absolutely no further anaesthetics were employed.

Throughout the operation my left hand rested on the patient's forehead, I gently closed her eyes, my right holding her two hands firmly, and I never stopped reinforcing her will, praising her courage, persuading her that she could scarcely feel any pain.

Mrs N. conducted herself admirably well, she didn't make the slightest movement, didn't let out a single cry, and when the operation was over she assured me that she had indeed suffered very little.

Three weeks later the patient left my clinic, perfectly cured, the plastic operation having been a complete success.

## OBS. 108.

LAPAROTOMY, TOTAL REMOVAL OF THE UTERUS AND ITS APPENDICES. SURGICAL ANAESTHESIA OBTAINED WITH A SMALL DOSE OF CHLOROFORM TOGETHER WITH HYPNOTIC SUGGESTION.

Miss M. H. aged 50 years, suffered from nervous symptoms of a hysterical kind treated by hypnotic suggestion. She fell into a deep sleep easily and realised perfectly suggestions regarding sensation, she didn't get to the state of somnambulism (Liébault's sixth degree).

For some years she had been suffering from profuse menorrhagia, probably caused by the presence of fibromyomas in the uterus. More recently the tumours had grown so much in volume that they were giving rise to serious secondary phenomena necessitating a radical operation.

Very much weakened by the repeated loss of blood, nervous in the extreme, the patient didn't seem to the surgeon to present the desired conditions for undergoing an operation — with the best chances of a cure — one so serious as a laparo-hysterectomy. Complications necessitating prolonged anaesthesia could occur, one point above all was the object of serious concern on the part of the surgeon, whether Miss M. H. could tolerate the chloroform. These preoccupations did not escape the notice of the patient. She summoned me and asked me to tell her if I thought that in her case suggestive anaesthesia could replace anaesthesia with chloroform. I replied that it was impossible for me to be sure since the idea of undergoing such a serious operation, which would capture so much of her awareness, meant that suggestion might not neutralise her pain.

However I proposed to combine the two procedures notably: chloroformisation and hypnotic suggestion. I undertook to give the chloroform while at the same time suggesting sleep and analgesia.

The patient and the surgeon were happy with this proposition and the operation was fixed for 3 May 1893.

Thanks to my preparatory suggestions the patient had a good night and went courageously into the operating theatre at the appointed time.

I got her to lie down and applied the mask moistened with a few drops of chloroform, addressing calming words to her all the time. Without a phase of excitement, the analgesia was produced almost instantaneously and the operation began. It lasted about an hour and gave no cause for concern. I estimated the quantity of narcotic employed at about 10 cc.

A quarter of an hour after the operation the patient woke up spontaneously, she was neither nauseated nor vomiting. Hypnotic suggestion constituted a serious adjunct to her convalescent treatment.

## OBS. 109.

PAINLESS EXTRACTION OF A TOOTH. SUGGESTIVE ANALGESIA.

Miss C. N. a very suggestible hysteric, good somnambulist, having been under my care for some time and ridded of some functional troubles, developed dental caries in the second molar on the right side of her lower jaw. The dentist that she consulted assured her that the decay was too advanced for him to be able to save the tooth. Having learnt that Miss C. N. was treated by hypnotism and knowing that she was disinclined to have a tooth extracted without narcotisation, the dentist suggested to the patient that she have the operation in my clinic under hypnotic anaesthesia. I gladly put myself at the disposal of the dentist and the patient's desire and we arranged the date and time of the operation.

At the appointed time, the dentist and Miss C. N. came to my room together where I was standing with my back turned whilst washing my hands. I asked the dentist to get on with his job. "Excuse me", he said, "but you first need to put Miss to sleep." "Certainly sir, it's done." " How…but?…" with those words the dentist looked at me enquiringly.

I turned towards him and addressing myself to the patient:

" Miss are you asleep yes or no?"

" Perfectly" she responded laughing. In fact she was standing in the middle of the room with her eyes closed.

"Would you allow this gentleman to extract your tooth?"

" But of course."

" The gentleman will hurt you?"

" Not in the least."

" You hear sir, go ahead if you would like to."

The dentist was dumbstruck, couldn't believe his eyes, proceeded with the operation. He removed the molar, without the patient showing the least sign of pain. The deed having been done, I took Miss C. N. to rinse her mouth and woke her up afterwards.

Complete amnesia.

## OBS. 110.

ANALGESIA BY SUGGESTION; PAINLESS EXTRACTION OF A TOOTH.

One of my easily hypnotisable patients who fell into a deep sleep, Miss M. P., suffered from a bad tooth. She wanted to go to her dentist the next day to have it removed. However, wishing to be rid of it without pain she asked me to put her to sleep and to suggest anaesthesia of the affected area for the following day. I put myself at her disposal and gave her the requested suggestion.

I saw the patient again several days afterwards. Informing me that everything had gone according to plan, she confirmed she had been perfectly calm at the dentist's and that he, having extracted her tooth, couldn't understand how she hadn't shown the least sign of suffering, when on other occasions she had always put up a frightening song and dance. When Miss M. P. explained that her analgesia was an effect of my suggestion, the dentist shrugged his shoulders and smiled incredulously.

ACKNOWLEDGEMENTS

Many thanks are due to Kate Wilson, Coralie Fong Wah, and Robin and Daphne Briggs.

www.ingramcontent.com/pod-product-compliance
Lightning Source LLC
Chambersburg PA
CBHW030607220526
45463CB00004B/1194